Essentials of Shock Management

Gil Joon Suh
Editor

Essentials of Shock Management

A Scenario-Based Approach

Springer

Editor
Gil Joon Suh
Department of Emergency Medicine
Seoul National University Hospital
Seoul
South Korea

ISBN 978-981-10-5405-1 ISBN 978-981-10-5406-8 (eBook)
https://doi.org/10.1007/978-981-10-5406-8

Library of Congress Control Number: 2018961688

This Springer imprint is published by the registered company Springer Nature Singapore Pte Ltd.
The registered company address is: 152 Beach Road, #21-01/04 Gateway East, Singapore 189721, Singapore

Preface

The initial management of shock in the real world, especially in the emergency department, requires a thorough understanding of pathophysiology, rapid assessment of shock, and comprehensive and timely treatment. There are a number of excellent textbooks for shock management. A traditional and ideal textbook-based approach is helpful for the management of simple and typical shock. However, the initial management of shock in the real world is not straightforward. A textbook-based approach which is based on symptoms, signs, and hemodynamic and laboratory parameters of classified typical shock has difficulties in solving complicated shock, which is often seen in the emergency department or ICU.

A scenario-based approach to shock is a new approach to shock management. In this approach, real shock cases which were seen in the emergency department are reconstructed into scenarios based on real-life experiences. It would be helpful to solve the complicated shock cases. In this respect, this book was written entirely by emergency physicians who have diverse experience in the management of the patients with different types of complicated shock in the emergency department.

This book is composed of three parts. The first part is the introduction which includes definition, classification, pathophysiology, diagnosis, and management of shock. In the second part, introduction, pathophysiology, initial approach and diagnosis, initial management, and future investigation according to the different types of shock—hemorrhagic, cardiogenic, obstructive, septic, and anaphylactic—are described. In the third part, a key part of this book, a scenario-based approach to a series of cases based on real-life experiences is given. Here, a narrative style and Q&A form are employed to vividly convey scenarios that may be encountered in clinical practice and to elucidate decision making in complex circumstances. A storytelling form of scenario will be very interesting and realistic because clinical presentation, underlying disease, and laboratory and radiologic findings are obtained from real patients. When readers experience difficulty in answering the questions, the earlier sections (first and second parts) can be consulted to identify the correct response.

Although this book was written by emergency physicians, it will be of great value in resuscitation and critical care. In particular, it will be very helpful for a novice or inexperienced person in emergency medicine, critical care medicine, or traumatology.

Seoul, South Korea Gil Joon Suh

Contents

Contributors

Han Sung Choi Department of Emergency Medicine, Kyung Hee University School of Medicine, Seoul, South Korea

Sung-Hyuk Choi Institute for Trauma Research, Korea University, Seoul, South Korea

Sung Phil Chung Department of Emergency Medicine, Gangnam Severance Hospital, Yonsei University College of Medicine, Seoul, South Korea

You Hwan Jo Department of Emergency Medicine, Seoul National University Bundang Hospital, Gyeonggi-do, South Korea

Joonghee Kim Department of Emergency Medicine, Seoul National University Bundang Hospital, Gyeonggi-do, South Korea

Kyung Su Kim Department of Emergency Medicine, Seoul National University Hospital, Seoul, South Korea

Kyuseok Kim Department of Emergency Medicine, Seoul National University Bundang Hospital, Gyeonggi-do, South Korea

Won Young Kim Department of Emergency Medicine, University of Ulsan College of Medicine, Asan Medical Center, Seoul, South Korea

Woon Yong Kwon Department of Emergency Medicine, Seoul National University College of Medicine, Seoul, South Korea

Hui Jai Lee Department of Emergency Medicine, Seoul Nation University – Seoul Metropolitan Government Boramae Medical Center, Seoul, South Korea

Jae Hyuk Lee Department of Emergency Medicine, Seoul National University Bundang Hospital, Gyeonggi-do, South Korea

Jonghwan Shin Department of Emergency Medicine, Seoul National University College of Medicine, Seoul, South Korea

Gil Joon Suh Department of Emergency Medicine, Seoul National University College of Medicine, Seoul, South Korea

Part I

Introduction

1 Introduction of Shock

Gil Joon Suh and Hui Jai Lee

1.1 Introduction

1.1.1 Definition of Shock

Traditionally shock was defined as an arterial hypotension resulting from impaired cardiac output, blood loss, or decreased vascular resistance. With development of the technology and the increase in understanding shock physiology, cell-level definition has been introduced. In this respect, shock is a state of circulatory failure to deliver sufficient oxygen to meet the demands of the tissues, that is, the imbalance between oxygen delivery and oxygen consumption in the tissues, which results in cellular dysoxia. One recent consensus meeting defined shock as "a life-threatening, generalized form of acute circulatory failure associated with inadequate oxygen utilization by the cells" [1].

G. J. Suh (✉)
Department of Emergency Medicine,
Seoul National University College of Medicine,
Seoul, South Korea
e-mail: suhgil@snu.ac.kr

H. J. Lee
Department of Emergency Medicine,
Seoul Nation University – Seoul Metropolitan
Government Boramae Medical Center,
Seoul, South Korea
e-mail: emdrlee@snu.ac.kr

1.1.2 Cellular Oxygen Delivery and Utilization

Oxygen is crucial for ATP production to maintain cellular metabolic function and homeostasis. Inadequate oxygen supplement cannot meet the oxygen demand and causes cellular injury.

In shock state, oxygen delivery (DO_2) is deceased and tissue oxygen consumption (VO_2) is increased. Imbalance between DO_2 and VO_2 is a key mechanism of the shock.

Restoration of tissue perfusion, prevention of cell damage, and maintenance of organ function are basic principles of shock management [1–6].

1.1.2.1 Tissue Oxygen Delivery

Tissue oxygen delivery is defined as a process to deliver arterial oxygenated blood to tissue. Arterial oxygen content (CaO_2) is determined by the amount of oxygen bound to hemoglobin (SaO_2) and dissolved oxygen in plasma.

Arterial oxygen content is described as follows:

$$CaO_2 = \frac{1.34 \times Hb \times SaO_2}{(\text{Hemoglobin} - \text{bound oxygen amount})} + \frac{0.0031 \times PaO_2}{(\text{Dissolved oxygen to plasma})}$$

G. J. Suh (ed.), *Essentials of Shock Management*, https://doi.org/10.1007/978-981-10-5406-8_1

Oxygen delivery to tissue (DO_2) can be expressed as a product of arterial oxygen content and cardiac output (CO).

Therefore, the equation for DO_2 is as follows:

$$DO_2 = CO \times CaO_2$$
$$= CO \times (1.34 \times Hb \times SaO_2 + 0.0031 \times PaO_2)$$

The amount of oxygen dissolved in plasma is so small relative to oxygen bound to hemoglobin that the dissolved oxygen in plasma has a limited role in tissue oxygen delivery.

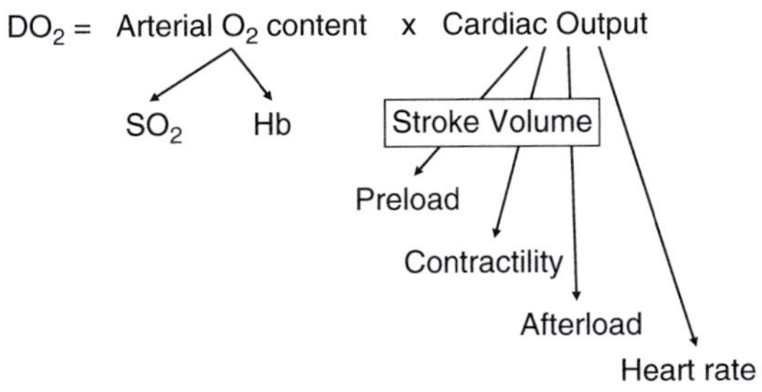

Fig. 1.1 Determinants of oxygen delivery. *DO_2* oxygen delivery, *SaO_2* oxygen saturation, *Hb* hemoglobin

Therefore, the equation for DO_2 can be simplified [7]:

$$DO_2 = CO \times (1.34 \times Hb \times SaO_2)$$

CO is the product of stroke volume (SV) and heart rate (HR).

SV is composed of three components: preload, myocardial contractility, and afterload.

Therefore, adequate CO, hemoglobin level, and oxygen saturation are essential (Fig. 1.1).

Tissue Oxygen Uptake

Tissue oxygen uptake means the amount of oxygen consumed by tissues and cannot be measured directly.

Instead, VO_2 is calculated from difference between the amount of oxygen supplement (DO_2) and amount of oxygen in returned venous blood (Fig. 1.2).

Venous oxygen content (CvO_2) can be expressed similarly to arterial oxygen content:

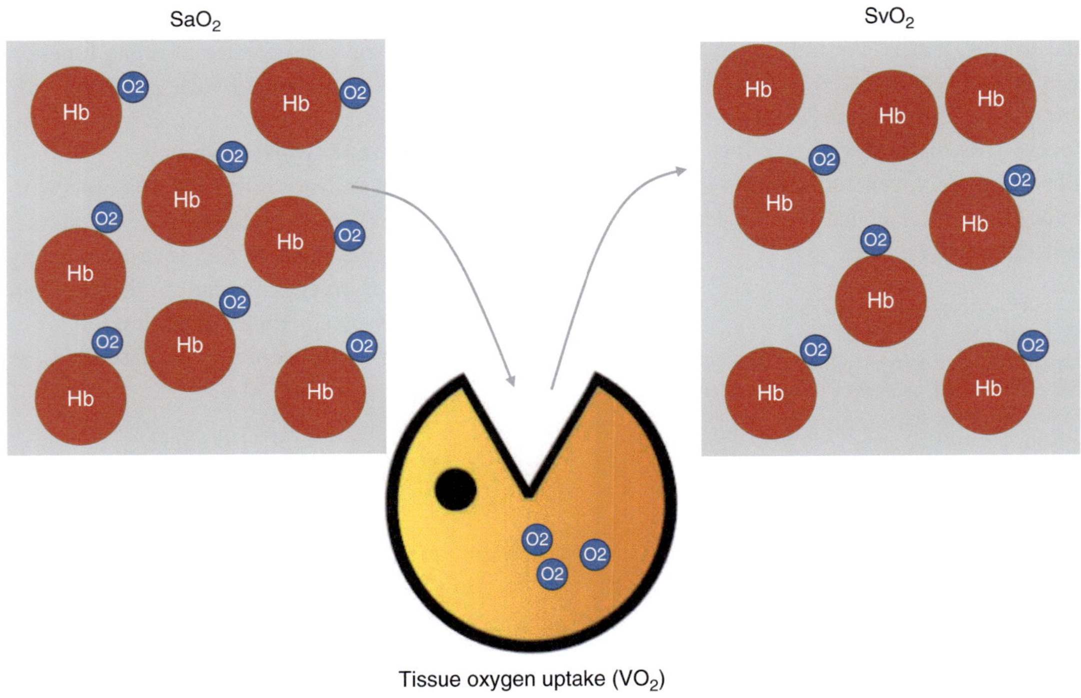

Fig. 1.2 Tissue oxygen uptake is calculated by difference between arterial oxygen saturation and venous oxygen saturation

$$CvO_2 = 1.34 \times Hb \times SvO_2$$
$$VO_2 = CO \times (CaO_2 - CvO_2)$$
$$= CO \times 1.34 \times Hb \times (SaO_2 - SvO_2)$$

SvO_2 means mixed venous oxygen saturation. It can be measured with pulmonary artery catheter. Because pulmonary artery catheterization is an invasive procedure, central venous oxygen saturation ($ScvO_2$) which can be drawn from central venous catheter can be used as a surrogate marker for SvO_2 [2]. However, substituting SvO_2 by $ScvO_2$ may be inappropriate because the difference between SvO_2 and $ScvO_2$ is variable in some critically ill patients [8, 9].

1.1.3 Epidemiology

The presence of the shock is usually risk factors of poor prognosis. According to a European multicenter trial, septic shock was the most common (62%) type of shock in the ICU, followed by cardiogenic (16%), hypovolemic (16%), distributive other than septic (4%), and obstructive shock (2%) [10].

1.2 Classification of Shock

Shock has been traditionally classified into four types: hypovolemic, cardiogenic, obstructive, and distributive shock (Table 1.1) [6, 11].

Hypovolemic shock occurs when circulating blood volume is decreased such as bleeding, dehydration, and gastrointestinal loss. Decreased circulating blood causes deceased preload, stroke volume, and cardiac output. Reduced cardiac output causes a compensatory increase in systemic vascular resistance.

Cardiogenic shock is caused by failure of cardiac pump function. Most common cause of cardiogenic shock is myocardial infarction. Other conditions including arrhythmia, cardiomyopathy, and valvular heart disease may decrease cardiac output.

Obstructive shock is caused by the anatomical or functional obstruction of cardiovascular flow system. It includes pulmonary embolism, pericardial tamponade, tension pneumothorax, and systemic arterial obstruction (large embolus, tumor metastasis, direct compression by adjacent tumor, aortic dissection, etc.).

Table 1.1 Type of shock

Type	Hemodynamic changes	Etiologies
Hypovolemic	Decreased preload Increased SVR Decreased CO	Hemorrhage, capillary leak, GI losses, burns
Cardiogenic	Increased preload Increased afterload Increased SVR Decreased CO	MI, dysrhythmia, heart failure, valvular disease
Obstructive	Decreased preload Increased SVR Decreased CO	PE, pericardial tamponade, tension pneumothorax, LV outlet obstruction
Distributive	Decreased preload Increased SVR Mixed CO	Septic shock, anaphylactic shock, neurogenic shock

CO cardiac output, *GI* gastrointestinal, *SVR* systemic vascular resistance, *MI* myocardial infarction, *PE* pulmonary embolism, *LV* left ventricle

Systemic vasodilation and secondary effective intravascular volume depletion result in distributive shock. Septic shock, the most common type of shock, is a kind of distributive shock. Neurogenic shock and anaphylaxis are also included in distributive shock [11, 12].

Several types of shock can coexist in a patient. For example, a patient with septic shock may be complicated by cardiogenic shock, which is caused by stress-induced cardiomyopathy.

1.3 Pathophysiology of Shock

Although there are various kinds of shock with many different clinical conditions, shock is a circulatory mismatch between tissue oxygen supply and tissue oxygen demand.

1.3.1 Vascular Response

For maintaining vital organ perfusion, several autonomic responses are activated.

Stimulation of carotid baroreceptor stretch reflex activates the sympathetic nervous system.

The activation of sympathetic nervous system increases heart rate and myocardial contractility and redistributes the blood flow from skin, skeletal muscles, kidney, and splanchnic organs to vital organs. Dominant autoregulatory control of blood flow spares cerebral and cardiac blood supply.

Release of vasoactive hormones increases the vascular tones. Antidiuretic hormone and activation of renin-angiotensin axis inhibit renal loss of sodium and water and help to maintain intravascular volume.

1.3.2 Microcirculatory Dysfunction

In normal condition, capillary perfusion is well maintained. In shock, however, reduced capillary density and perfusion are shown. Shock is also characterized by endothelial cell damage, glycocalyx alteration, activation of coagulation, microthrombi formation, and leukocytes and red blood cell alteration, which lead to microcirculatory dysfunction [5, 13].

1.3.3 Cellular Injury

Under the normal condition, 38 adenosine triphosphates (ATP) are produced via aerobic glycolysis and TCA cycle.

In shock, however, pyruvate cannot enter into the TCA cycle due to insufficient oxygen delivery (anaerobic glycolysis), which results in only two ATP production. In this process, pyruvate is converted into lactate in cell which is released into circulation (Fig. 1.3).

When cellular hypoperfusion persists, cellular energy stores are rapidly decreased due to inadequate ATP regeneration. After ATP depletion, energy-dependent cellular systems are impaired, cellular homeostasis is threatened, and the breakdown of ultrastructure occurs.

Inappropriate activation of systemic inflammation also causes cellular injures, which leads to multiple organ dysfunction (Fig. 1.4).

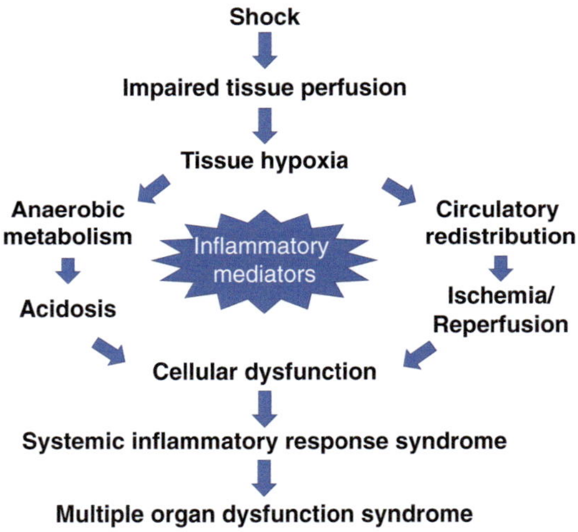

Fig. 1.4 Pathophysiology of shock

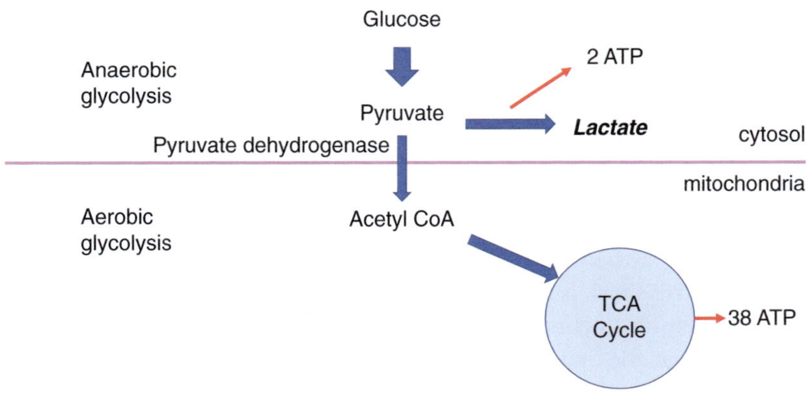

Fig. 1.3 Glycolysis pathway. Without oxygen, efficiency of ATP generation is markedly decreased. Lactate is a by-product of anaerobic glycolysis pathway. *ATP* adenosine triphosphate, *TCA* tricarboxylic acid

1.4 Diagnosis of Shock

Diagnosis of shock should be based on comprehensive considerations of clinical, hemodynamic, and biochemical features.

1.4.1 Clinical Features

Tissue hypoperfusion in shock state can cause various kinds of organ dysfunctions. A comprehensive and detailed clinical assessment for the early detection and acute management is required.

1.4.1.1 General Appearance

Shock is a life-threatening condition and stressful reactions such as anxiety, irritability, and agitation can be observed. Diaphoresis, pale skin, and mottled skin suggesting tissue hypoperfusion may be present. Capillary refill time more than 2 s can be used as a surrogate marker of tissue hypoperfusion.

1.4.1.2 Central Nerve System

Patients with shock often present with various symptoms of CNS dysfunction. Visual disturbance, dizziness, syncope, agitation, mental status, delirium, or seizure can be present. Decreased mentality or presence of delirium is associated with increased mortality [14, 15].

1.4.1.3 Respiratory System

Tachypnea is a component of the systemic inflammatory response, and common symptom of shock. Medullary hypoperfusion stimulates respiratory center and augments respiratory effort. Increased workload of breathing combined with persistent hypoperfusion to respiratory muscles eventually causes respiratory muscle fatigue and leads to early respiratory failure. ARDS can develop as a consequence of inflammatory responses induced by shock.

1.4.1.4 Kidney

Renal hypoperfusion and oliguria cause ischemic renal damage. The extent of acute kidney injury is variable in shock. There are a number of clinical tools for the assessment of acute kidney injury. Among them, RIFLE criteria and KIDIGO definition are most commonly used (Tables 1.2 and 1.3) [16, 17].

1.4.1.5 Gastrointestinal Tract

Bowel mucosa is injured by hypoperfusion, splanchnic vasoconstriction caused by the redistribution of blood, and inflammatory insult. Bowel injury causes the destruction of mucosal

Table 1.2 RIFLE criteria [16]

	GFR criteria	Urine output criteria
Risk	Increased serum creatinine × 1.5 or GFR decrease >25%	UO < 0.5 mL/kg/h × 6 h
Injury	Increased serum creatinine × 2 or GFR decrease >50%	UO < 0.5 mL/kg/h × 12 h
Failure	Increased serum creatinine × 3 or GFR decrease >70% or serum creatinine 4 mg/dL (acute rise 0.5 mg/dL)	UO < 0.3 mL/kg/h × 24 h or anuria × 12 h
Loss	Persistent AKI Complete loss of kidney function >4 weeks	
ESRD	End-stage kidney disease (>3 months)	

GFR glomerular filtration rate, *UO* urine output

Table 1.3 KIDIGO definition of AKI [17]

AKI is defined as any of the following: - Increase in SCr by ≥0.3 mg/dL within 48 h - Increase in SCr to ≥1.5 times baseline, which is known or presumed to have occurred within the prior 7 days - Urine volume <0.5 mL/kg/h for 6 h
Stage 1 - Increase in SCr by 1.5–1.9 times baseline - Increase in sSCr by ≥0.3 mg/dL - Urine output <0.5 mL/kg/h for 6–12 h Stage 2 - Increase in SCr by 2.0–2.9 times baseline OR - Urine output <0.5 mL/kg/h for ≥12 h Stage 3 - Increase in SCr by 3.0 times baseline - Increase in SCr to 4.0 mg/dL - Initiation of renal replacement therapy - In patients <18 years, decrease in eGFR to 35 mL/min/1.73 m^2 - Urine output <0.3 mL/kg/h for ≥24 h - Anuria for ≥12 h

AKI acute kidney injury, *SCr* serum creatinine, *eGFR* estimated glomerular filtration rate

integrity, leading to bacterial translocation and inflammation-mediated injury [18].

1.4.1.6 Liver

Liver is vulnerable to hypoperfusion and tissue hypoxia. Increase in hepatic enzymes including transaminase and lactate dehydrogenase is common. The synthesis of coagulation factors is impaired by hepatic dysfunction.

1.4.1.7 Hematologic Disorder

Anemia can develop due to direct blood loss (e.g., hemorrhagic shock, acute gastric mucosal bleeding), myelosuppression, and hemolysis. Thrombocytopenia, coagulopathy, and disseminated intravascular coagulation (DIC) can develop. As mentioned above, hepatic injury can worsen the coagulation dysfunction.

1.4.1.8 Metabolic Disorder

Circulatory shock is a stressful event and sympathetic activity is stimulated in the early phase. An increase in release of catecholamine, cortisol, and glucagon and decrease in insulin release can be shown. As a result, hyperglycemia can be shown in the early phase of shock. In advanced stage of shock, hypoglycemia can be present due to glycogen depletion or failure of hepatic glucose synthesis.

Fatty acids are increased early in shock period. However, fatty acids are decreased in the late phase due to hypoperfusion to adipose tissue.

1.4.1.9 Clinical Scoring Systems

Several clinical scoring systems can be used for the assessment of circulatory shock for critically ill patients. Acute Physiology and Chronic Health Evaluation (APACHE) scores (II, III, IV), Simplified Acute Physiology Score (SAPS II), and Sequential Organ Failure Assessment (SOFA) score are commonly used and can be applied to the circulatory shock patients (Table 1.4) [19–23].

1.4.2 Hemodynamic Features

1.4.2.1 Blood Pressure and Heart Rate Monitoring

Blood Pressure

A decrease in cardiac output causes vasoconstriction, leading to decreased peripheral perfusion to maintain arterial pressure. However, preserved blood pressure due to vasoconstric-

Table 1.4 Sequential Organ Failure Assessment (SOFA) score

	0	1	2	3	4
Respiratory PaO_2/FiO_2 (mmHg)	>400	≤400	≤300	≤200 and mechanically ventilated	≤100 and mechanically ventilated
Coagulation Platelet (×10³/μL)	>150	≤150	≤100	≤50	≤20
Liver Bilirubin (μmol/L)	1.2	1.2–1.9	2.0–5.9	6.0–11.9	>12.0
Cardiovascular Hypotension	No hypotension	MAP <70 mmHg	Dopamine <5 or dobutamine (any)	Dopamine >5, epinephrine ≤0.1, or norepinephrine ≤0.1	Dopamine >15, epinephrine >0.1, or norepinephrine >0.1
Central nerve system GCS scale	15	13–14	10–12	6–9	<6
Renal Creatinine (μmol/L) or urine output (mL/d)	<1.2	1.2–1.9	2.0–3.4	3.5–4.9 or <500	>5.0 or <200

Catecholamine doses = μg/kg/min
FiO_2 fraction of inspired oxygen, *MAP* mean arterial pressure, *GCS* Glasgow coma score

tion may be associated with inadequate tissue perfusion, such as decreased central venous oxygen saturation ($ScvO_2$) and increase in blood lactate. Although the presence of hypotension is essential in the diagnosis of septic shock, it is not necessary to define the other types of shock [1, 5, 6].

Indirect measurement of blood pressure is often inaccurate in severe shock status and insertion of arterial catheter should be considered. Mean arterial pressure (MAP) reflects cardiac output better than systolic or diastolic pressure, and is often used as the guidance of shock treatment. The radial artery is commonly used. Femoral, brachial, axillary, or dorsalis artery can be used [7, 24, 25].

Heart Rate

Heart rate is the vital component of the cardiac output. According to the ATLS classification, class II hemorrhage (estimated blood loss 15–30%) showed a tachycardia of >100 beats/min, but normal systolic blood pressure. It means that heart rate is a more sensitive indicator than blood pressure in the early phase of hemorrhage shock [26].

Shock Index

Shock index is HR/systolic BP ratio. It reflects better circulatory status than heart rate or blood pressure alone. Normal ratio is between 0.5 and 0.8. Increased shock index is related with poor outcomes of traumatic or septic shock [27, 28]. Shock index also has predictive value for cardiogenic shock [29, 30].

1.4.2.2 Central Venous Pressure (CVP)

CVP, a direct right atrial pressure, is an indicator of blood volume status. Low CVP (<4 mmHg) in critically ill patient indicates severe volume depletion such as dehydration or acute blood loss requiring volume resuscitation (Table 1.4). However, because CVP is affected by multiple factors including venous tone, intravascular volume, right ventricular contractility, or pulmonary hypertension, CVP-guided shock treatment is no longer recommended. CVP should be interpreted together with other hemodynamic parameters [25, 31].

1.4.2.3 Cardiac Output

Pulmonary Artery Catheter

Pulmonary artery catheter is a flow-directed catheter with balloon tip. It is inserted through the jugular, subclavian, or femoral vein and advanced to the right atrium, right ventricle, and pulmonary artery. It measures cardiac output with thermodilution method and has been the reference method for measuring cardiac output in shock states. However, no randomized trial showed benefit of pulmonary artery catheter placement in critically ill patients [32–37]. Because of its invasiveness, routine placement of pulmonary artery catheter is not recommended. However, pulmonary artery catheter can measure accurate right atrial pressure and pulmonary artery pressure; it may be particularly useful in cases of shock associated with the right-sided heart failure, pulmonary hypertension, and/or difficult ARDS (Tables 1.5 and 1.6) [24].

Table 1.5 Hemodynamic characteristics of the shock

	Preload			
	Pulmonary capillary wedge pressure	Central venous pressure	Cardiac output	Systemic vascular resistance
Hypovolemic	Decreased	Decreased	Decreased	Increased
Cardiogenic	Increased	Increased	Decreased	Increased
Obstructive	Decreased	Decreased	Decreased	Increased
Distributive				
Early	Decreased	Decreased	Increased	Decreased
Late	Increased	Increased	Decreased	Increased

Table 1.6 Hemodynamic monitoring of shock

Preload	Cardiac contractility	Afterload	Cardiac output	Cellular oxygenation
Pulmonary artery catheter CVP Echocardiography Transpulmonary thermodilution systems	Echocardiography Transpulmonary thermodilution systems	Transpulmonary thermodilution systems	Pulmonary artery catheter Transpulmonary thermodilution systems Bioimpedance	NIRS Videomicroscopy techniques

Transpulmonary Thermodilution

Although less invasive than pulmonary artery catheter, transpulmonary thermodilution method also requires the insertion of central venous catheter and arterial catheter for the measurement of cardiac output. This method has been shown to be equivalent in accuracy to invasive pulmonary artery thermodilution technique [24]. Cardiac output is intermittently measured via the thermodilution technique using cold saline infusion. Compared to pulmonary artery catheter, the difference is that cold saline is injected not into the right atrium but into a central vein and changes of the blood temperature are detected not in the pulmonary artery but in a systemic artery. Cardiac output measured by this technique has shown a good agreement with that using pulmonary artery catheter in critically ill patients [38].

Continuous cardiac output is measured by the arterial pulse contour analysis. Global end diastolic volume, intrathoracic blood volume, extravascular lung water volume, pulmonary blood volume, pulmonary vascular permeability index, global ejection fraction, contractility, and systemic vascular resistance can also be measured or calculated with this device. Currently commercially available devices are PiCCO and VolumeView/EV1000 system [29].

Transpulmonary Dye Dilution

In this method, lithium, instead of saline, is injected through vein (central or peripheral) and measures changes of the blood temperature in a peripheral artery using specialized sensor probe [39].

LiDCO system is a commercially available transpulmonary dye dilution device.

Ultrasound Flow Dilution (The Costatus System)

After cold saline infusion, this method measures cardiac output with ultrasound velocity and blood flow change instead of thermodilution. It requires a primed extracorporeal arteriovenous tube set (AV loop). Two ultrasound flow-dilution sensors are placed on the arterial and venous ends and provide ultrasound dilution curve through which cardiac output can be calculated [40].

Echocardiography

Echocardiography is an important diagnostic method for evaluation of cardiac status. Nowadays its use is increasing for the management of acute and critically ill patients using bedside sonographic devices [41].

Cardiac output can be measured using pulsed-wave Doppler velocity in the left ventricular outflow tract. Comprehensive sonographic approach can help differential diagnosis of shock. It can help rapidly recognize the physical status of patients, and select therapeutic options [42–44]. Moreover, repeated evaluations can be done easily and help evaluating response to the treatment and help.

Pulse Contour and Pulse Pressure Analysis

Several kinds of devices are developed to estimate cardiac output from an arterial pressure waveform signal. This method reflects changes of cardiac output well in stable patients. However, accuracy is not guaranteed if vascular tone change occurs, which is common in the shock state or when vasoactive drugs are used [45]. Several devices including FloTrac/Vigileo and LiDCOrapid/pulseCO are available.

Bioimpedance

Blood has a relatively low electrical resistance and intrathoracic blood volume change causes significant impedance changes of thoracic cavity. This method detects voltage changes using skin electrode and postulates blood volume changes during cardiac cycle and cardiac output. Any conditions which can affect intrathoracic fluid, such as pleural effusion or lung edema, influence the result of bioimpedance method. This is not a calibrated method and accuracy in measuring cardiac output is questionable [24].

1.4.2.4 Microcirculatory and Tissue Perfusion Monitoring

Near-Infrared Spectroscopy

Near-infrared spectroscopy (NIRS) is a noninvasive technique used for observing real-time changes in tissue oxygenation. Several studies showed prognostic ability of NIRS in septic shock [46–48].

Videomicroscopy Techniques

These handheld microscopic camera devices can visualize capillaries, venules, and even movement of erythrocyte. These methods can help evaluating microcirculatory status. Sublingual microcirculation is usually evaluated in humans. Vessel perfusion status, quality of capillary flow, and presence of non-perfused area are often evaluated [49].

Sidestream dark-field (SDF) or incident dark-field (IDF) technique is used. The orthogonal polarization spectral (OPS) imaging device has been replaced by newer devices based on SDF or IDF imaging [49].

1.4.2.5 Other Indirect Methods

Gastric Tonometry

Tissue hypoxia causes lactate production and metabolic acidosis. Gastrointestinal mucosa is vulnerable to hypoxic injury, easily influenced by remote organ injuries. Stomach can be easily assessed with nasogastric tube. Gastric tonometry measures gastric mucosal CO_2 and calculates gastric mucosal pH assuming that arterial bicarbonate and mucosal bicarbonate are equal. Tissue hypoperfusion results in reduction of gastric mucosal pH. However, this assumption is not correct and mucosal bicarbonate and pH are influenced by various conditions; results should be interpreted with caution [50].

1.5 Management of Shock

1.5.1 Initial Management

1.5.1.1 Airway and Breathing

Airway management is important in patients with shock. Early intubation should be considered in case of respiratory distress, hypoxemia, severe acidosis, and decreased mentality and when airway protection is threatened.

Increased work of breathing increases the oxygen consumption of the respiratory muscles. Decreased work of breathing with intubation and adequate sedation can help improve the tissue oxygen delivery.

Positive pressure ventilation can reduce preload and worsen the hypotension or cause cardiovascular collapse. Volume resuscitation and vasopressor support (if indicated) should be performed before positive ventilation.

1.5.1.2 Fluid Resuscitation

Fluid resuscitation should be started for restoring microvascular circulation when there is evidence of shock.

Initial fluid should be started with isotonic crystalloid. However endovascular permeability is increased in shock state; risk of acute edema with unwanted consequence is high when excessive fluid is infused. Careful monitoring of fluid responsiveness is required. Volume status, cardiac output, blood pressure, and tissue perfusion status should be evaluated repeatedly [6, 25].

1.5.1.3 Fluid Responsiveness

Although adequate volume restoration is a key to the treatment of the shock, excessive fluid resuscitation causes tissue edema, endothelial injury, and impairment of tissue perfusion. Volume overload is related with the poor prognosis of shock patients. Static parameters such as CVP or PAWP or global end diastolic volume is no longer useful, and they alone should not be used for predicting fluid responsiveness. Dynamic parameters such as pulse pressure variation (PPV), stroke volume variation (SVV), or velocity time integral (VTI) are better than static variables to predict fluid responsiveness (Table 1.7) [1, 51].

Pulse Pressure or Stroke Volume Variation

In case of volume depletion, the cardiac output is influenced by the change of the thoracic pressure. During inspiration period, the thoracic pressure rises and right ventricular and left ventricular preload decrease.

These parameters are usually checked during mechanical ventilation and adequate amount of tidal volume ($\geq$7–8 mL/kg). In cases of spontaneous breathing, low tidal volume, or cardiac arrhythmia, pulse pressure or stroke volume variations cannot be assessed accurately. Changes more than 12% are considered as volume-sensitive status (sensitivity 79–84%, specificity 84%) [52].

Table 1.7 Methods for evaluating fluid responsiveness

Static parameter	Dynamic parameter
Central venous pressure Pulmonary capillary wedge pressure	Pulse pressure variation Stroke volume variation Inferior vena cava variation Response to passive leg raising Changes in cardiac output following passive leg raising

Static parameters no longer recommended for evaluation of fluid responsiveness

Passive Leg Raising

Passive leg raising causes movement of blood pooled in the lower extremity to the central circulation. Maximizing the response, the patient has semirecumbent position and change to leg-raising position (Fig. 1.5). During the procedure, direct measurement of cardiac output should be performed.

Positive fluid balance can be expected with 10% or more changes in cardiac output (sensitivity 88%, specificity 92%) [51, 52].

1.5.1.4 Vasopressor

Vasopressor should be started after adequate fluid resuscitation except anaphylactic shock (epinephrine should be injected first) or cardiac arrest. There is no universal optimal target blood pressure. In hemorrhagic shock, hypotensive resuscitation is recommended before definite bleeding control. However, blood pressure target in traumatic brain injury should be higher for maintaining cerebral perfusion pressure [1, 6, 25].

Most vasopressors improve the blood pressure by increasing the vascular resistance and can result in decrease in the capillary perfusion.

1.5.2 Restoring Tissue Perfusion

1.5.2.1 Lactate

Lactate is the product of tissue anaerobic metabolism. Increased blood level reflects the tissue hypoxia and hypoperfusion, and is particularly a useful tool to identify patients with septic shock. If the lactate level has not decreased by 10–20%

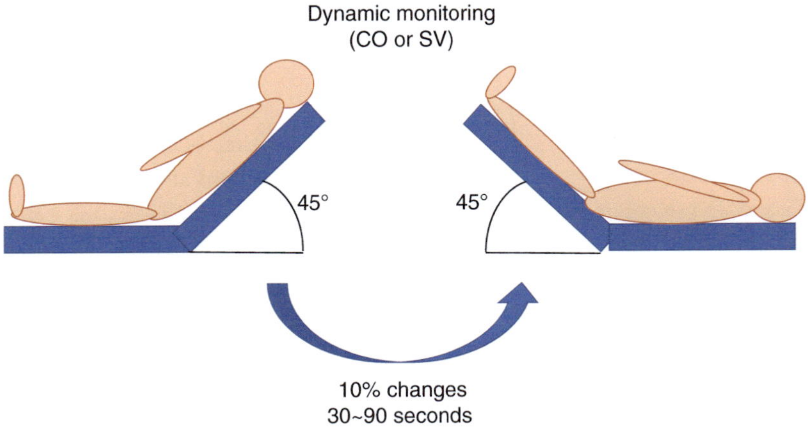

Fig. 1.5 Passive leg-raising test

within 2 h after resuscitation, additional interventions to improve tissue oxygenation should be implemented [1, 25].

1.5.2.2 Specific Treatment of Causes of Shock

Etiology of shock is various and accurate methods to maintain tissue perfusion can be different according to the etiology of shock. Causes of shock should be sought aggressively and etiology-specific treatment should be started promptly. These will be discussed in later parts of this book.

1.6 Summary

- Shock is an imbalance between tissue oxygen supplement and utilization, not just a state of low blood pressure.
- Fundamental of shock treatment is restoration of tissue oxygenation and tissue function.
- Close monitoring of perfusion status and supportive care for organ dysfunctions is important.
- Find specific etiologies of shock and treat them.

References

1. Cecconi M, De Backer D, Antonelli M, Beale R, Bakker J, Hofer C, et al. Consensus on circulatory shock and hemodynamic monitoring. Task force of the European Society of Intensive Care Medicine. Intensive Care Med. 2014;40(12):1795–815.
2. Rivers E, Nguyen B, Havstad S, Ressler J, Muzzin A, Knoblich B, et al. Early goal-directed therapy in the treatment of severe sepsis and septic shock. N Engl J Med. 2001;345(19):1368–77.
3. Singer M, Deutschman CS, Seymour CW, Shankar-Hari M, Annane D, Bauer M, et al. The third international consensus definitions for sepsis and septic shock (sepsis-3). JAMA. 2016;315(8):801–10.
4. Suess EM, Pinsky MR. Hemodynamic monitoring for the evaluation and treatment of shock: what is the current state of the art? Semin Respir Crit Care Med. 2015;36(6):890–8.
5. De Backer D, Orbegozo Cortes D, Donadello K, Vincent J-L. Pathophysiology of microcirculatory dysfunction and the pathogenesis of septic shock. Virulence. 2014;5(1):73–9.
6. Vincent JL, De Backer D. Circulatory shock. N Engl J Med. 2013;369(18):1726–34.
7. Marino PL. The ICU book. 4th ed. Philadelphia: Wolters Kluwer Health/Lippincott Williams & Wilkins; 2014.
8. Chawla LS, Zia H, Gutierrez G, Katz NM, Seneff MG, Shah M. Lack of equivalence between central and mixed venous oxygen saturation. Chest. 2004;126(6):1891–6.
9. Walley KR. Use of central venous oxygen saturation to guide therapy. Am J Respir Crit Care Med. 2011;184(5):514–20.
10. De Backer D, Biston P, Devriendt J, Madl C, Chochrad D, Aldecoa C, et al. Comparison of dopamine and norepinephrine in the treatment of shock. N Engl J Med. 2010;362(9):779–89.
11. Weil MH, Shubin H. Proposed reclassification of shock states with special reference to distributive defects. Adv Exp Med Biol. 1971;23:13–23.
12. Landry DW, Oliver JA. The pathogenesis of vasodilatory shock. N Engl J Med. 2001;345(8):588–95.
13. Ashruf JF, Bruining HA, Ince C. New insights into the pathophysiology of cardiogenic shock: the role of the microcirculation. Curr Opin Crit Care. 2013;19(5):381–6.
14. Ely E, Shintani A, Truman B, et al. Delirium as a predictor of mortality in mechanically ventilated patients in the intensive care unit. JAMA. 2004;291(14):1753–62.
15. Kataja A, Tarvasmaki T, Lassus J, Kober L, Sionis A, Spinar J, et al. Altered mental status predicts mortality in cardiogenic shock—results from the CardShock study. Eur Heart J Acute Cardiovasc Care. 2018;7(1):38–44. https://doi.org/10.1177/2048872617702505.
16. Bellomo R, Ronco C, Kellum JA, Mehta RL, Palevsky P. Acute renal failure—definition, outcome measures, animal models, fluid therapy and information technology needs: the Second International Consensus Conference of the Acute Dialysis Quality Initiative (ADQI) Group. Crit Care. 2004;8(4):R204–12.
17. Palevsky PM, Liu KD, Brophy PD, Chawla LS, Parikh CR, Thakar CV, et al. KDOQI US Commentary on the 2012 KDIGO Clinical Practice Guideline for Acute Kidney Injury. Am J Kidney Dis. 2013;61(5):649–72.
18. Deitch EA. The role of intestinal barrier failure and bacterial translocation in the development of systemic infection and multiple organ failure. Arch Surg. 1990;125(3):403–4.
19. Knaus WA, Draper EA, Wagner DP, Zimmerman JE. APACHE II: a severity of disease classification system. Crit Care Med. 1985;13(10):818–29.
20. Knaus WA, Wagner DP, Draper EA, Zimmerman JE, Bergner M, Bastos PG, et al. The APACHE III prognostic system. Risk prediction of hospital mortality for critically ill hospitalized adults. Chest. 1991;100(6):1619–36.

21. Zimmerman JE, Kramer AA, McNair DS, Malila FM. Acute physiology and chronic health evaluation (APACHE) IV: hospital mortality assessment for today's critically ill patients. Crit Care Med. 2006;34(5):1297–310.
22. Le Gall JR, Lemeshow S, Saulnier F. A new simplified acute physiology score (SAPS II) based on a European/North American multicenter study. JAMA. 1993;270(24):2957–63.
23. Vincent JL, Moreno R, Takala J, Willatts S, De Mendonca A, Bruining H, et al. The SOFA (Sepsis-related Organ Failure Assessment) score to describe organ dysfunction/failure. On behalf of the Working Group on Sepsis-Related Problems of the European Society of Intensive Care Medicine. Intensive Care Med. 1996;22(7):707–10.
24. Sakka SG. Hemodynamic Monitoring in the Critically Ill Patient – Current Status and Perspective. Front Med. 2015;2:44.
25. Rhodes A, Evans LE, Alhazzani W, Levy MM, Antonelli M, Ferrer R, et al. Surviving sepsis campaign: International Guidelines for Management of Sepsis and Septic Shock: 2016. Crit Care Med. 2017;45(3):486–552.
26. Surgeons ACo. Advanced trauma life support for doctors–student course manual. 8th ed. Chicago: American College of Surgeons; 2008.
27. Haider AA, Azim A, Rhee P, Kulvatunyou N, Ibraheem K, Tang A, et al. Substituting systolic blood pressure with shock index in the National Trauma Triage Protocol. J Trauma Acute Care Surg. 2016;81(6):1136–41.
28. Tseng J, Nugent K. Utility of the shock index in patients with sepsis. Am J Med Sci. 2015;349(6):531–5.
29. Yu T, Tian C, Song J, He D, Sun Z, Sun Z. Derivation and validation of shock index as a parameter for predicting long-term prognosis in patients with acute coronary syndrome. Sci Rep. 2017;7(1):11929.
30. Zhang X, Wang Z, Wang Z, Fang M, Shu Z. The prognostic value of shock index for the outcomes of acute myocardial infarction patients: a systematic review and meta-analysis. Medicine. 2017;96(38):e8014.
31. Boyd JH, Forbes J, Nakada TA, Walley KR, Russell JA. Fluid resuscitation in septic shock: a positive fluid balance and elevated central venous pressure are associated with increased mortality. Crit Care Med. 2011;39(2):259–65.
32. Connors AF Jr, Speroff T, Dawson NV, Thomas C, Harrell FE Jr, Wagner D, et al. The effectiveness of right heart catheterization in the initial care of critically ill patients. Supp Invest JAMA. 1996;276(11):889–97.
33. Harvey S, Harrison DA, Singer M, Ashcroft J, Jones CM, Elbourne D, et al. Assessment of the clinical effectiveness of pulmonary artery catheters in management of patients in intensive care (PAC-Man): a randomised controlled trial. Lancet. 2005;366(9484):472–7.
34. Rajaram SS, Desai NK, Kalra A, Gajera M, Cavanaugh SK, Brampton W, et al. Pulmonary artery catheters for adult patients in intensive care. Cochrane Database Syst Rev. 2013;2013(2):Cd003408.
35. Richard C, Warszawski J, Anguel N, Deye N, Combes A, Barnoud D, et al. Early use of the pulmonary artery catheter and outcomes in patients with shock and acute respiratory distress syndrome: a randomized controlled trial. JAMA. 2003;290(20):2713–20.
36. Sandham JD, Hull RD, Brant RF, Knox L, Pineo GF, Doig CJ, et al. A randomized, controlled trial of the use of pulmonary-artery catheters in high-risk surgical patients. N Engl J Med. 2003;348(1):5–14.
37. Wheeler AP, Bernard GR, Thompson BT, Schoenfeld D, Wiedemann HP, de Boisblanc B, et al. Pulmonary-artery versus central venous catheter to guide treatment of acute lung injury. N Engl J Med. 2006;354(21):2213–24.
38. Monnet X, Teboul JL. Transpulmonary thermodilution: advantages and limits. Crit Care. 2017;21(1):147.
39. Jonas MM, Tanser SJ. Lithium dilution measurement of cardiac output and arterial pulse waveform analysis: an indicator dilution calibrated beat-by-beat system for continuous estimation of cardiac output. Curr Opin Crit Care. 2002;8(3):257–61.
40. Crittendon I, Dreyer WJ, Decker JA, Kim JJ. Ultrasound dilution: an accurate means of determining cardiac output in children. Pediatr Crit Care Med. 2012;13(1):42–6.
41. Levitov A, Frankel HL, Blaivas M, Kirkpatrick AW, Su E, Evans D, et al. Guidelines for the appropriate use of bedside general and cardiac ultrasonography in the evaluation of critically ill patients-Part II: cardiac ultrasonography. Crit Care Med. 2016;44(6):1206–27.
42. Frankel HL, Kirkpatrick AW, Elbarbary M, Blaivas M, Desai H, Evans D, et al. Guidelines for the appropriate use of bedside general and cardiac ultrasonography in the evaluation of critically ill patients-Part I: general ultrasonography. Crit Care Med. 2015;43(11):2479–502.
43. Shokoohi H, Boniface KS, Pourmand A, Liu YT, Davison DL, Hawkins KD, et al. Bedside ultrasound reduces diagnostic uncertainty and guides resuscitation in patients with undifferentiated hypotension. Crit Care Med. 2015;43(12):2562–9.
44. Ahn JH, Jeon J, Toh H-C, Noble VE, Kim JS, Kim YS, et al. SEARCH 8Es: a novel point of care ultrasound protocol for patients with chest pain, dyspnea or symptomatic hypotension in the emergency department. PLoS One. 2017;12(3):e0174581.
45. Cecconi M, Rhodes A. Pulse pressure analysis: to make a long story short. Crit Care. 2010;14(4):175.
46. Shapiro NI, Arnold R, Sherwin R, O'Connor J, Najarro G, Singh S, et al. The association of near-infrared spectroscopy-derived tissue oxygenation measurements with sepsis syndromes, organ dysfunction and mortality in emergency department patients with sepsis. Crit Care. 2011;15(5):R223.
47. Masip J, Mesquida J, Luengo C, Gili G, Goma G, Ferrer R, et al. Near-infrared spectroscopy StO2 monitoring to assess the therapeutic effect of drotrecogin alfa (activated) on microcirculation in patients with

severe sepsis or septic shock. Ann Intensive Care. 2013;3(1):30.
48. Marin-Corral J, Claverias L, Bodi M, Pascual S, Dubin A, Gea J, et al. Prognostic value of brachioradialis muscle oxygen saturation index and vascular occlusion test in septic shock patients. Med Int. 2016;40(4):208–15.
49. Massey MJ, Shapiro NI. A guide to human in vivo microcirculatory flow image analysis. Crit Care. 2016;20:35.
50. Heard SO. Gastric tonometry*: the hemodynamic monitor of choice (pro). Chest. 2003;123(5, Supplement):469S–74S.
51. Monnet X, Marik PE, Teboul JL. Prediction of fluid responsiveness: an update. Ann Intensive Care. 2016;6(1):111.
52. Bentzer P, Griesdale DE, Boyd J, MacLean K, Sirounis D, Ayas NT. Will this hemodynamically unstable patient respond to a bolus of intravenous fluids? JAMA. 2016;316(12):1298–309.

Part II

Types of Shock

Hemorrhagic Shock

2

You Hwan Jo and Sung-Hyuk Choi

2.1 Introduction

Hypovolemic shock is defined as a life-threatening, generalized form of acute circulatory failure associated with inadequate oxygen utilization by the cells due to hemorrhage, dehydration, and so on. Hypovolemic shock is the second most common shock and mortality rate is still high [1]. Hemorrhagic shock is the most serious type of hypovolemic shock and we are focusing on the hemorrhagic shock, especially traumatic shock, in this chapter. Trauma accounts for 10% of deaths worldwide, and the most common cause of death between 1 and 44 years [2].

2.2 Pathophysiology

Hemorrhagic shock is a state in which the circulation is unable to deliver sufficient oxygen to meet the demands of the tissues, resulting in cellular dysfunction that leads to organ dysfunction and death. Hypovolemia by blood loss stimulates the compensatory responses for baroreceptor which detects volume loss, and chemoreceptor which detects hypoxia to maintain blood pressure and cardiac output [3]. In addition, it causes the immune responses from the production of a protein and nonprotein mediators at the site of injury [4].

The compensatory reactions such as the cardiovascular response, the neuroendocrine response, and the immunologic and inflammatory response happen variously. Changes in cardiovascular function cause vasoconstriction and increase of myocardial contractility due to increases in α_1, β_1-adrenegic receptors to stimulation of sympathetic nerves. In the neuroendocrine responses, hemorrhage increases cortisol and vasopressin, resulting in hyperglycemia and intestinal ischemia due to mesenteric vasoconstriction. However, persistent hemorrhage stops the compensatory reactions and causes uptake of interstitial volume to intercellular space due to cell membrane dysfunction, resulting in the cell edema.

The function of the host immune system after hypovolemic shock is related to alterations in the production of mediators, such as tumor necrosis factor (TNF)-α, interleukin (IL)-1, IL-2, PGE_2 (prostaglandin), and IL-6, considered part of body's response to inflammation. In the cellular aspects of hemorrhagic shock, polymorphonuclear neutrophils (PMNs) play an important role in host defense response to the initial reaction of the inflammatory reaction, but

Y. H. Jo (✉)
Department of Emergency Medicine, Seoul National University Bundang Hospital, Gyeonggi-do, South Korea
e-mail: drakejo@snubh.org

S.-H. Choi
Institute for Trauma Research, Korea University, Seoul, South Korea
e-mail: kuedchoi@korea.ac.kr

G. J. Suh (ed.), *Essentials of Shock Management*, https://doi.org/10.1007/978-981-10-5406-8_2

also result in an adverse effect due to production of the reactive oxygen radicals (ROS), such as superoxide$^-$, hydrogen peroxide, and production of proteolytic enzymes. This PMN acts with vascular endothelial cells to increase the vascular permeability and reduce oxidative phosphorylation by mitochondria and loss of adenosine triphosphate (ATP) due to the hypoxic respiration of the cells, resulting in interruption of exchange in cell membrane, cell edema, and cell death. The T lymphocyte is most important in the role of the immune response to the mechanism of multiple-organ failure. In the event of a shock, the function of the lymphocytes is known to be related to the reduction in the decrease in IL-2. These cellular and microcirculatory changes have significant physiologic importance in the ability of the organism to recover from hemorrhagic shock.

The lethal triad of acidosis, hypothermia, and coagulopathy is commonly seen in patients with severe hemorrhagic shock (Fig. 2.1 [5]). Each factor in triad influences the other factors, and the patients with this lethal triad show high mortality in spite of aggressive management.

Hemorrhage induces tissue hypoperfusion and increased production of lactic acid which results in metabolic acidosis. In addition, aggressive fluid resuscitation with unbalanced crystalloid such as 0.9% sodium chloride solution could also induce hyperchloremic acidosis. Acidosis induces impairment of coagulation cascade characterized by prolongation of clot formation time and reduction of clot strength and decreased myocardial performance, resulting in tissue hypoperfusion and acidosis [6]. Hypothermia is induced by environmental exposure, massive bleeding, fluid resuscitation, and administration of sedative drugs. Hypothermia could induce platelet dysfunction, destabilization of coagulation factors, and increase in fibrinolytic activity [7].

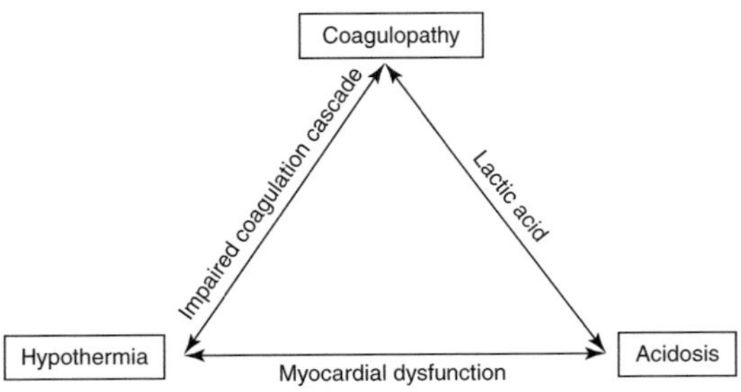

Fig. 2.1 Lethal triad of hemorrhagic shock

The importance of the early diagnosis and prevention of coagulopathy has increased significantly in recent years. Endogenous factors related with coagulopathy are endogenous anticoagulation, fibrinogen depletion, hyperfibrinolysis and fibrinolytic shutdown, platelet dysfunction, and endothelial dysfunction [8]. Coagulopathy could be worsened by several factors such as acidosis, hypothermia, anemia, and anticoagulants/antiplatelets.

2.3 Initial Approach and Diagnosis

Initial assessment of the severity of the patient and identification of the source of bleeding are crucial for the patient with hemorrhagic shock. Several classifications of hemorrhagic shock, imaging techniques, and laboratory tests are currently used for this purpose.

2.3.1 Clinical Assessment

The clinical manifestation of hemorrhagic shock is variable. It depends on the source of bleeding, rate, and volume of bleeding as well as the patient's physiologic status, underlying diseases, and medications being taken. Although traditional hemodynamic response to hemorrhage includes hypotension, tachycardia, and narrow pulse pressure, it varies between the patients and there are no absolute criteria reflecting the severity of hemorrhagic shock.

2.3.1.1 Classification of Hemorrhagic Shock

The classification of hemorrhage into four classes based on the initial clinical signs such as vital signs, mental status, and urine output was traditionally introduced and a useful

Table 2.1 Estimated blood loss based on the clinical signs

	Class I	Class II	Class III	Class IV
Blood loss (mL)	Up to 750	750–1500	1500–2000	>2000
Blood loss (%)[a]	Up to 15	15–30	30–40	>40
Pulse rate (beat/min)	<100	100–120	120–140	>140
Blood pressure	Normal	Normal	Decreased	Decreased
Pulse pressure	Normal or increased	Decreased	Decreased	Decreased
Respiratory rate (breath/min)	14–20	20–30	30–40	>35
Urine output (mL/h)	>30	20–30	5–15	Negligible
Mental status	Slightly anxious	Mildly anxious	Anxious, confused	Confused, lethargic
Fluid replacement	Crystalloid	Crystalloid	Crystalloid and blood	Crystalloid and blood

[a]For a 70 kg male patients

method for estimating the percentage of blood volume loss [9]. The estimated blood volume of normal adults is approximately 7% of body weight, and a 70 kg male has approximately 5 L of circulating blood volume (Table 2.1). There is variability in estimating blood volume, the blood volume of obese adult calculated based on the ideal body weight not on the actual body weight to prevent overestimation.

2.3.1.2 Responses to Initial Fluid Resuscitation

Patient's response to fluid resuscitation is an important factor for determination of subsequent treatment such as blood transfusion and intervention. Therefore, another classification was based on the patient's response to initial fluid resuscitation [9] (Table 2.2).

2.3.1.3 Score Systems

Several score systems have been introduced to predict the risk of hemorrhagic shock and the probability of massive transfusion. For example, the shock index is calculated as heart rate divided by systolic blood pressure and the TASH score (Trauma Associated Severe Hemorrhage) included seven parameters such as systolic blood pressure, hemoglobin, intra-abdominal fluid, complex long bone and/or pelvic fractures, heart rate, base excess, and gender [10]. However, these scores have not been validated well and have not been widely used yet.

Table 2.2 Responses to initial fluid resuscitation in trauma patients

	Rapid response	Transient response	Minimal to no response
Vital signs	Return to normal	Transient improvement	Remain abnormal
Estimated blood loss	Minimal (10–20%)	Moderate and ongoing (20–40%)	Severe (>40%)
Need for more crystalloid	Low	Low to moderate	Moderate as bridge to transfusion
Need for blood	Low	Moderate to high	Immediate
Blood preparation	Type and cross-match	Type specific	Emergency blood release
Need for operative intervention	Possibly	Likely	Highly likely
Early presence of surgeon	Yes	Yes	Yes

[a]Isotonic crystalloid solution, 2000 mL in adults and 20 mL/kg in children

2.3.2 Assessment of the Source of Bleeding

2.3.2.1 Identified Source of Bleeding

The source of bleeding in hemorrhagic shock may be sometimes obvious. In traumatic shock, penetrating trauma such as stab wounds or gunshot wounds usually has more obvious source of bleeding than blunt trauma and requires surgical bleeding control. In nontraumatic hemorrhagic shock, the approximate source of bleeding could be determined by the patient's symptoms such as hematemesis, hematuria, and vaginal bleeding. If a source of bleeding is identified, immediate procedures for bleeding control should be considered unless initial resuscitation is successful.

2.3.2.2 Unidentified Source of Bleeding

In contrast, a patient without obvious source of bleeding should undergo further investigation. In traumatic shock, early diagnostic imaging techniques such as ultrasonography or contrast-enhanced computed tomography (CT) are recommended for the detection of free fluid in patients with torso trauma [11].

Ultrasonography is a rapid, noninvasive imaging technique for detection of intra-abdominal fluid and can be performed in bedside without moving the patients. Extended focused assessment with sonography for trauma (eFAST) was introduced for trauma as a screening test for blood in the pericardium, abdominal cavity, or pleural space, and also for a pneumothorax. The six areas that are examined are subcostal (subxiphoid), RUQ (hepatorenal recess), LUQ (perisplenic space), pelvis, and thorax (Fig. 2.2).

Ultrasonography has been reported to have high specificity but relatively low sensitivity for the detection of intra-abdominal fluid [12–14]. Therefore, a positive finding in the ultrasonography suggests hemoperitoneum, but an initial negative finding cannot exclude hemoperitoneum and should perform serial ultrasonography or further imaging technique such as CT scan. The CT scan has been widely used to detect the source of bleeding in patients with hemorrhagic shock in both trauma and non-trauma, and the usefulness of the CT scan has been well known. Recently, multi-detector CT (MDCT) may require less than 30 s for scanning the whole body, and the usefulness of the CT scan has been well known [15, 16]. In addition, contrast-enhanced CT scan could detect active bleeding more accurately than non-enhanced CT scan [17, 18]. In contrast, diagnostic peritoneal lavage, one of the traditional diagnostic techniques, is rarely used when ultrasonography or CT is available.

In summary, if a patient has an obvious source of bleeding, immediate procedures for bleeding control should be performed, while if the source of bleeding is unidentified, further diagnostic techniques such as ultrasonography and contrast-enhanced MDCT should be performed.

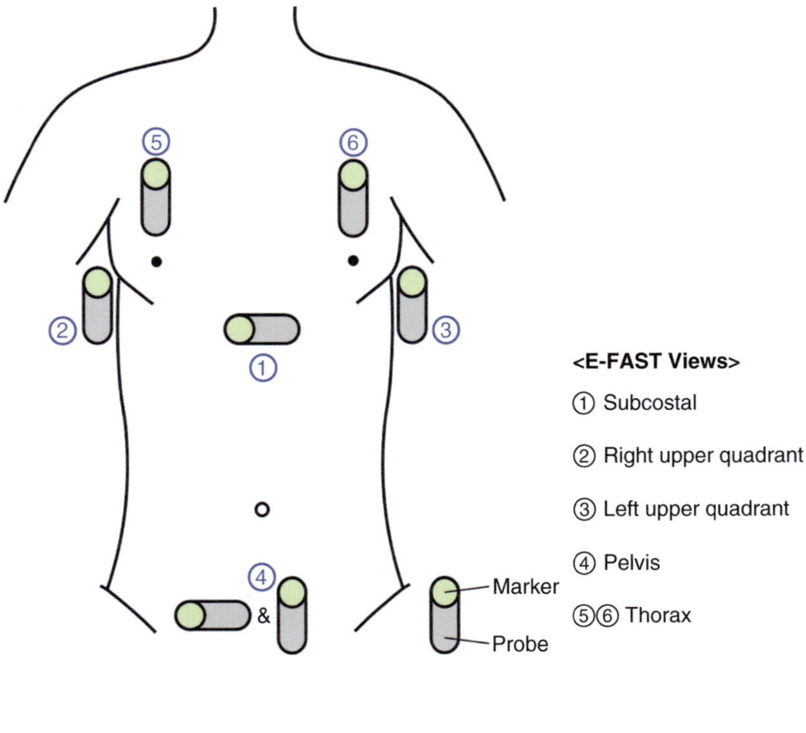

Fig. 2.2 Extended focused assessment with sonography for trauma (eFAST)

2.3.3 Laboratory Tests

Laboratory tests are a part of diagnostic workup for patients with hemorrhagic shock. They can help assess the condition and severity of the patient and identify the patients who may require aggressive diagnostic and therapeutic interventions. There are many laboratory tests that are necessary to the patient with hemorrhagic shock. In this part, we are focusing on the hematocrit, lactate, base deficit, and tests for coagulation.

2.3.3.1 Hemoglobin (Hb) and Hematocrit (Hct)

Hb and Hct are considered a basic test for hemorrhagic shock, but the diagnostic values of Hb and Hct have been debated. Low initial Hb is a marker of severe bleeding, but initial Hb and Hct may not reflect the volume of bleeding because patient bleeds whole blood and movement of fluids from interstitial space requires time [11]. In addition, initial fluid resuscitation and transfusion also influence the Hb and Hct. Therefore, serial measurements of hematocrit rather than single initial measurement could help assess the volume of hemorrhage.

2.3.3.2 Lactate

Lactate concentration is elevated by anaerobic glycolysis and it is a marker of tissue hypoperfusion. The role of lactate and lactate clearance was reported many times and it has been reported that lactate concentration was associated with mortality rate in trauma [19, 20].

2.3.3.3 Base Deficit

Base deficit also reflects metabolic acidosis by tissue hypoperfusion. Base deficit either from arterial or venous blood decreases in hemorrhagic shock, and it was associated with patient's outcome as with lactate concentration [21]. In addition, some authors reported that the base deficit was superior to pH for predicting outcome in trauma [22].

2.3.3.4 Conventional Coagulation Tests

Coagulopathy is a key feature of hemorrhagic shock, so measurement of coagulation is an important diagnostic test. Conventional monitoring of coagulation includes prothrombin time (PT), activated partial thromboplastin time (aPTT), and fibrinogen and platelet counts, and these tests remain the most widely used methods for the diagnosis of coagulopathy. Cutoff values for these tests may be different between the institutions. However, it has been reported that these conventional tests were not associated with outcome because these tests could reflect early coagulopathy in hemorrhagic shock [23, 24]. In other words, conventional coagulation tests may be normal despite the ongoing coagulopathy.

2.3.3.5 Viscoelastic Methods

To overcome the shortcomings of the conventional tests, viscoelastic methods such as thromboelastography (TEG) and rotational thromboelastometry (ROTEM) have been introduced and increasingly used in hemorrhagic shock. Although the values between two devices are not interchangeable due to different methods of assessment and definition of variables, similarities of information on clot formation kinetics and clot strength can be found. The most important variables are clotting time, clot formation/kinetics, clot strengthening, amplitude/maximal firmness, and lysis (Fig. 2.3 and Table 2.3) [25, 26].

In trauma, viscoelastic methods were used not only for identifying the trauma-induced coagulopathy but also for viscoelastic method-based treatment protocol in the trauma-induced coagulopathy and massive transfusion. It was reported that viscoelastic method-based protocol reduced mortality [27, 28].

In summary, serial measurements of hematocrit, lactate, base deficit, and monitoring of coagulation with conventional tests and viscoelastic methods are essential for diagnosis and guiding treatment in hemorrhagic shock.

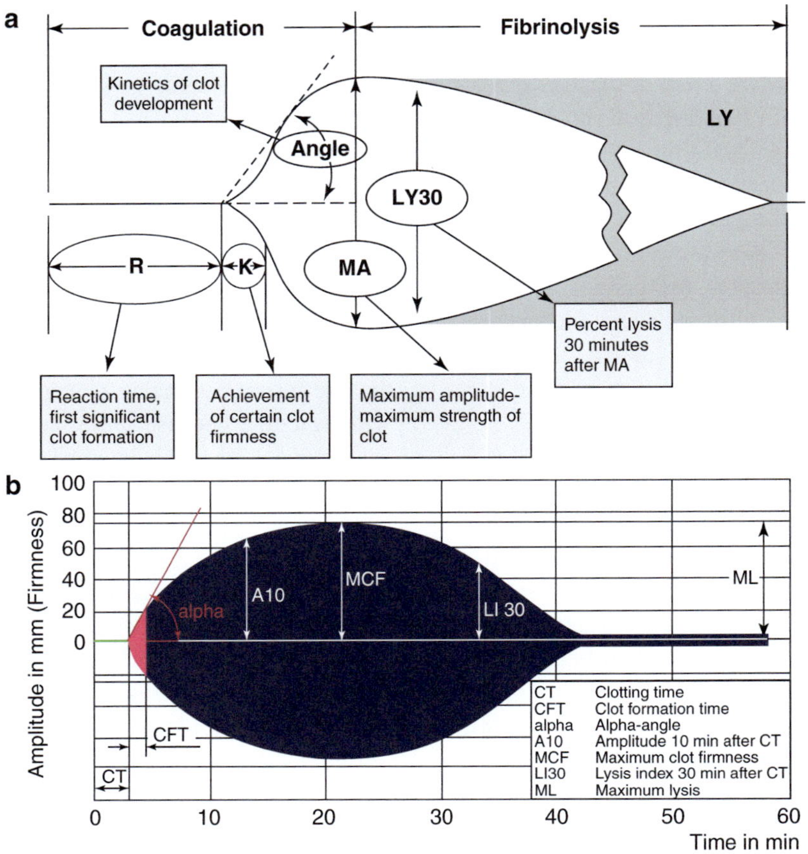

Fig. 2.3 Thromboelastography (TEG) and rotational thromboelastometry (ROTEM)

Table 2.3 Variables in thromboelastography (TEG) and rotational thromboelastometry (ROTEM)

Variables	TEG	ROTEM
Clotting time (2 mm amplitude)	R (reaction time) Normal (citrate/kaolin): 3–8 min	CT (clotting time) Normal (EXTEM): 42–74 s Normal (INTEM): 137–246 s
Clot formation/ kinetics (20 mm amplitude)	K (kinetics) Normal (citrate/kaolin): 1–3 min	CFT (clot formation time) Normal (EXTEM): 46–148 s Normal (INTEM): 40–100 s
Clot strengthening (angle of clot formation)	Alfa angle (slope between r and k points) Normal (citrate/kaolin): 55–78	Alfa angle (slope of tangent at 2 mm amplitude) Normal (EXTEM): 63–81 Normal (INTEM): 71–82
Amplitude/maximal firmness	MA (maximal amplitude) Normal (citrate/kaolin): 51–69 mm	MCF (maximum clot firmness) Normal (EXTEM): 49–71 mm Normal (INTEM): 52–72 mm Normal (FIBTEM): 9–25 mm A5, A10, etc.: amplitudes at dedicated time points predicting the final clot firmness
Lysis	CL30, CL60, CL	LI30, LI60, ML

2.4 Initial Management of Hemorrhagic Shock

The goal of initial resuscitation for hemorrhagic shock is to arrest ongoing bleeding, to restore the effective circulating blood volume, and to restore tissue perfusion. Management protocol of hemorrhagic shock has developed based on the treatment of trauma patients. There was a concept of damage control surgery (DCS) as a surgical approach to the trauma, and this has been expanded to the early management of trauma patients as damage control resuscitation (DCR) [29]. Early recognition of the patients with high risk and prevention of lethal triad of coagulopathy, hypothermia, and acidosis are main purposes of the DCR. The components in the DCR are described in Table 2.4 [30, 31]. In this part, we discuss the key management of hemorrhagic shock.

2.4.1 Target of Blood Pressure

In the traditional treatment of hemorrhagic shock, rapid and large volume of crystalloid was used to restore normal hemodynamics. However, this traditional fluid resuscitation may cause dislodgement of blood clots on the bleeding sites, dilution of coagulation factors, and hypothermia of the shock patient [11]. In addition, it may exacerbate the hemorrhagic shock-induced inflammatory responses and induce immune dysregulation. As a different concept from the traditional resuscitation, permissive hypotension was introduced. It is a concept of low-volume fluid resuscitation and it avoids the adverse effects of traditional resuscitation while maintaining tissue perfusion for a short period [32]. Several retrospective and prospective studies reported the benefit of the hypotensive resuscitation strategy in the aspect of survival rate, coagulopathy, and volume of blood product transfusion [33, 34]. In addition, brief periods (60–90 min) of permissive hypotension did not significantly increase the risk of irreversible end-organ damage or mortality. Therefore, a target systolic blood pressure of 80–90 mmHg is recommended currently in the initial resuscitation phase [11]. However, higher target of blood pressure (mean arterial pressure ≥80 mmHg) should be maintained in the hypotensive patient with traumatic brain injury for restoring cerebral perfusion pressure [35]. In addition, hypotensive strategy should be applied with caution in the elderly or the patient with chronic hypertension.

Table 2.4 Damage control resuscitation

Rapid recognition of coagulopathy and shock
Permissive hypotension
Rapid surgical control of bleeding
Prevention/treatment of hypothermia, acidosis, and hypocalcemia
Avoidance of hemodilution induced by aggressive intravenous fluid
Transfusion of red blood cells (RBC):plasma:platelets in a high unit ratio (>1:2) or reconstituted whole blood in a 1:1:1 unit ratio
Early and appropriate use of coagulation factor concentrates
The use of fresh RBCs and whole blood when available

2.4.2 Type of Fluids

Fluid resuscitation is the first step to restore intravascular volume and tissue perfusion in hemorrhagic shock, and many types of fluids are currently available. However, it is unclear whether crystalloids or colloids should be used in hemorrhagic shock, and which fluid is better than the other.

2.4.2.1 Colloids

Hydroxyethyl starch (HES) a synthetic colloid and the effect of HES has been investigated in the hemorrhagic shock. One study reported that HES (130/0.4) improved lactate clearance and showed less renal injury in penetrating injury [36]. However, another study did not demonstrate the beneficial effects of HES, but rather increased bleeding volume, and showed harmful effect [37]. HES may decrease the von Willebrand factor, interfere with the polymerization of fibrinogen and platelet function, and exert deleterious kidney effect, so HES is not recommended in critically ill patients.

Albumin is recommended in patients with sepsis for fluid resuscitation, but the use of albumin instead of saline showed higher tendency of mortality in trauma, especially in patients with traumatic brain injury [38, 39]. Therefore, albumin is not recommended in trauma.

In the meta-analysis, colloids did not demonstrate any beneficial effect [40]. Colloids are more expensive than crystalloids and there has been no supporting evidence for use of colloids in hemorrhagic shock yet, so crystalloids are recommended initially for the management of hemorrhagic shock [11].

2.4.2.2 Crystalloids

Crystalloids include saline solution, Hartmann solution, Ringer's lactate or acetate solution, plasma-lyte solution, and so on. The 0.9% sodium chloride solution has been used widely, but this may increase chloride concentration, acidosis, and incidence of acute kidney injury [41]. It was reported that a balanced electrolyte solution caused less hyperchloremia and improved acid-base status [42]. Among the crystalloids, hypotonic solutions such as Hartmann solution and Ringer's lactate solution are not recommended in hemorrhagic shock with traumatic brain injury because they could worsen cerebral edema [11].

Potential benefits of the hypertonic saline are restoration of intravascular volume with a small volume, reduction of intracranial pressure in traumatic brain injury, and modulation of the inflammatory responses. In penetrating injury with hemorrhagic shock, hypertonic saline showed improving survival rate [43]. However, another study and a meta-analysis did not demonstrate any beneficial effect of hypertonic saline in hemorrhagic shock [40, 44].

In summary, colloids did not demonstrate any beneficial effect, and crystalloids are recommended as initial fluid for the patients with hemorrhagic shock.

2.4.3 Vasopressors and Inotropes

In hemorrhagic shock, dysregulated sympathetic response may develop because of sedation and systemic inflammatory response syndrome, and nitric oxide production. Fluid resuscitation is the first step to restore intravascular volume and hemodynamic variables, and vasopressors may be required in the life-threatening hypotension despite fluid resuscitation.

Norepinephrine is a sympathomimetic agent with vasoconstrictive effect. Norepinephrine stimulates alpha-adrenergic receptor and induces arterial vasoconstriction. In addition, norepinephrine also induces splanchnic venoconstriction which shifts splanchnic blood to the systemic circulation [45]. The effect of vasopressors including norepinephrine and vasopressin has been investigated, but human study is not sufficient. However, in patients with hemorrhagic shock with poor response to fluid resuscitation, vasopressors are recommended to maintain blood pressure. Myocardial dysfunction may also develop in hemorrhagic shock and inotropes such as dobutamine could be used in the presence of myocardia dysfunction [11].

2.4.4 Temperature Control

Hypothermia induces platelet dysfunction, coagulation factor dysfunction, enzyme inhibition, and fibrinolysis, and is associated with acidosis, hypotension, and coagulopathy in hemorrhagic shock [46, 47]. Hypothermia in hemorrhagic shock results in high morbidity and mortality, and patients with hypothermia requires more blood transfusion [48, 49].

Hypothermia in hemorrhagic shock should be prevented and warm the patients with hypothermia using measures such as removing wet clothing, covering the patient, infusion of warm fluid, forced warm air, and rewarming devices [11].

2.4.5 Massive Transfusion

2.4.5.1 Definition of Massive Transfusion

Traditional definition of massive transfusion was the transfusion of ten or more units of red blood cells (RBCs) within 24 h, but this definition has not been validated and has many problems. For example, a patient who receives 9 units of RBC within 4 h and ultimately dies in 6 h does not meet the traditional definition. Several definitions of massive transfusion have been introduced, such as ≥10 units of RBC within 6 h, ≥3 units of RBC per h, and ≥50% of blood volume within 4 h in adult, but all of these definitions cannot include the victims who die early for severe hemorrhagic shock. Therefore, other terms such as substantial bleeding, resuscitation intensity, and critical administration threshold have been introduced instead of massive transfusion [50–52]. Briefly, substantial bleeding included ≥1 unit of RBC within 2 h and ≥5 units of RBC or death within 4 h, and resuscitation intensity included numbers of units (fluid and blood products) infused within 30 min of arrival, and critical administration threshold included ≥3 units of RBC in any 1 h within 24 h [53].

2.4.5.2 Prediction of Massive Transfusion

Prediction of the need for massive transfusion is difficult. Many scoring systems have been developed and the scores included various variables such as hypotension, tachycardia, presence of intra-abdominal fluid, mechanism of injury, and laboratory results.

One of the validated scoring systems is the assessment of blood consumption (ABC) score [54]. The ABC score included four parameters of penetrating torso injury, systolic blood pressure ≤90 mmHg, heart rate ≥120 bpm, and positive focused assessment with sonography for trauma (FAST). Each parameter is given one point and a score of two or more warrants massive transfusion protocol. The ABC score is simple and does not include laboratory results, and many institutions have used this. The American College of Surgeons Trauma Quality Improvement Program Massive Transfusion in Trauma Guidelines recommended that the criteria to trigger the activation of massive transfusion protocol should include one of the following parameters: ABC score ≥2, persistent hemodynamic instability, active bleeding requiring operation or angioembolization, and blood transfusion in the trauma bay (https://www.facs.org/w/media/files/quality%20programs/trauma/tqip/massive%20transfusion%20in%20trauma%20guildelines.ashx).

2.4.5.3 Protocol of Initial Transfusion

There are still conflicting opinions about the optimal ratio of RBC to plasma or platelet. As the use of rapid point-of-care test (POCT) of coagulation is increasing, transfusion of the selected blood components according to the results of the coagulation test is possible. Actually, rapid POCT is not available in many institutions, so initial management with blood components with a predefined ratio may be reasonable. Several retrospective studies demonstrated the benefit of higher ratios of plasma and platelet to RBC [55, 56]. In a prospective cohort study, higher ratios of plasma and platelet to RBC showed decreased mortality [57]. However, the optimal ratio was controversial because of the possible survival bias which means survivors may receive more plasma and platelet than non-survivors [58]. In addition, complications related with transfusion such as transfusion-related acute lung injury and volume overload are also a concern. In a recent prospective randomized study, there was no difference in mortality at 24 h or 30 days. However higher ratio group achieved hemostasis and fewer experienced death due to exsanguination, and the rate of complication was similar [59].

Another controversy is the use of plasma for replacement of fibrinogen. Fibrinogen depletion is known to be associated with poor outcome and administration of fibrinogen could improve survival [60].

In the European guidelines, at least 1:2 ratio of plasma to RBC, or fibrinogen concentrate and RBC according to hemoglobin level, is recommended [11]. The target hemoglobin level is recommended as 7–9 g/dL.

2.4.6 Pharmacologic Agents and Blood Products

2.4.6.1 Tranexamic Acid

Tranexamic acid is a synthetic lysine analogue and an antifibrinolytic agent as a competitive inhibitor of plasminogen. In a prospective cohort study, tranexamic acid reduced organ failure and mortality in traumatic shock patients [61]. A prospective randomized study showed that early administration of tranexamic acid reduced mortality in trauma patients with shock and the rate of thrombosis was not increased with the use of tranexamic acid [62]. In the subgroup analysis, administration of tranexamic acid after 3 h from injury increased death due to bleeding [63]. The effect of tranexamic acid has been reported in various surgical conditions such as cardiovascular surgery and orthopedic surgery. Recently, early administration of tranexamic acid also demonstrated reduced mortality in postpartum hemorrhage [64]. The recommended dose is a loading dose of 1 g over 10 min, followed by infusion of 1 g over 8 h, and tranexamic acid is not recommended more than 3 h after injury.

2.4.6.2 Calcium

Hypocalcemia is a common complication of massive transfusion. Low ionized calcium concentration was associated with increased mortality and massive transfusion [65, 66]. Therefore, ionized calcium concentration should be monitored and maintained within normal range.

2.4.6.3 Blood Products and Their Derivatives

Many blood products and their derivatives are currently used for the treatment of hemorrhagic shock. The brief indications and doses based on the current management guideline for trauma is summarized in the Table 2.5 [11].

When patients who have been treated with factor Xa inhibitors such as rivaroxaban, apixaban, or edoxaban suffered from major bleeding, tranexamic acid and prothrombin complex concentrate are recommended. In patients treated with thrombin inhibitors such as dabigatran, idarucizumab (5 g intravenously) or tranexamic acid and prothrombin complex concentrate are recommended [11].

Table 2.5 Current recommendation of further resuscitation for traumatic shock patients

	Indication	Initial dose
Fresh frozen plasma	1. PT and aPTT ≥1.5 times the normal control	1:1 or 1:2 ratio to RBC
Fibrinogen or cryoprecipitate	1. Functional fibrinogen deficit 2. Plasma fibrinogen <1.5–2.0 g/L	3–4 g of fibrinogen 15–20 units of cryoprecipitate
Platelets	1. General: Platelet count <50 × 10^9/L 2. Ongoing bleeding: Platelet count <100 × 10^9/L 3. Patients treated with antiplatelet agents	4–6 units or one apheresis
Prothrombin complex concentrate	1. Vitamin K-dependent oral anticoagulant 2. Patients treated with novel oral anticoagulant	25–50 IU/kg
Recombinant-activated coagulant factor VII	Continuing of major bleeding despite other attempts	Various (20–140 μg/kg)

2.4.6.4 Pharmacologic Agents for Gastrointestinal Hemorrhage

Upper gastrointestinal hemorrhage is a serious medical condition and it sometimes induces hemorrhagic shock. General management of the upper gastrointestinal hemorrhage is not different with that of traumatic shock. Several pharmacologic agents have been used for the treatment of the non-variceal hemorrhage such as proton pump inhibitors (PPIs), histamine H_2 receptor antagonist (H2RA), somatostatin analogue, and tranexamic acid. Among these agents, PPIs are associated with decreased all-cause mortality, rebleeding, and need for surgery. In contrast, H2RA and somatostatin analogue did not show any beneficial effect [67]. In the variceal hemorrhage, terlipressin and somatostatin analogues are currently used [68].

2.4.7 Bleeding Control

Bleeding control is the most important step for the management of hemorrhagic shock. The methods of bleeding control are various according to the mechanism of bleeding (trauma vs. non-trauma) and anatomical source of bleeding.

2.4.7.1 Tourniquet and Pelvic Stabilization

When life-threatening bleeding occurs from extremity injuries, a tourniquet should be applied and be left until surgical bleeding control is achieved. In patients with pelvic ring disruption, immediate pelvic ring closure with a pelvic binder, a pelvic C-clamp, or a bed sheet should be applied for stabilization of pelvic ring. In addition, pelvic packing can be used to decrease ongoing bleeding from the pelvic fracture.

2.4.7.2 Angiographic Embolization

Angiographic embolization is widely used for the management of hemorrhagic shock in trauma and non-trauma for controlling arterial bleeding. However angiographic embolization should not delay surgical bleeding control and multidisciplinary approach is important.

2.4.7.3 Resuscitative Endovascular Balloon Occlusion of the Aorta (REBOA)

REBOA has been used in a variety of clinical settings for patients with life-threatening hemorrhagic shock (Fig. 2.4). It may decrease early death from hemorrhagic shock and should be applied with subsequent surgery or angiographic embolization. The evidence for the usefulness of REBOA is weak and there is no definite protocol [69]. Therefore, a prospective study is warranted to investigate the role of REBOA in hemorrhagic shock.

2.4.7.4 Local Hemostatic Agents

Various local hemostatic agents are available for the control of hemorrhage. These local hemostatic

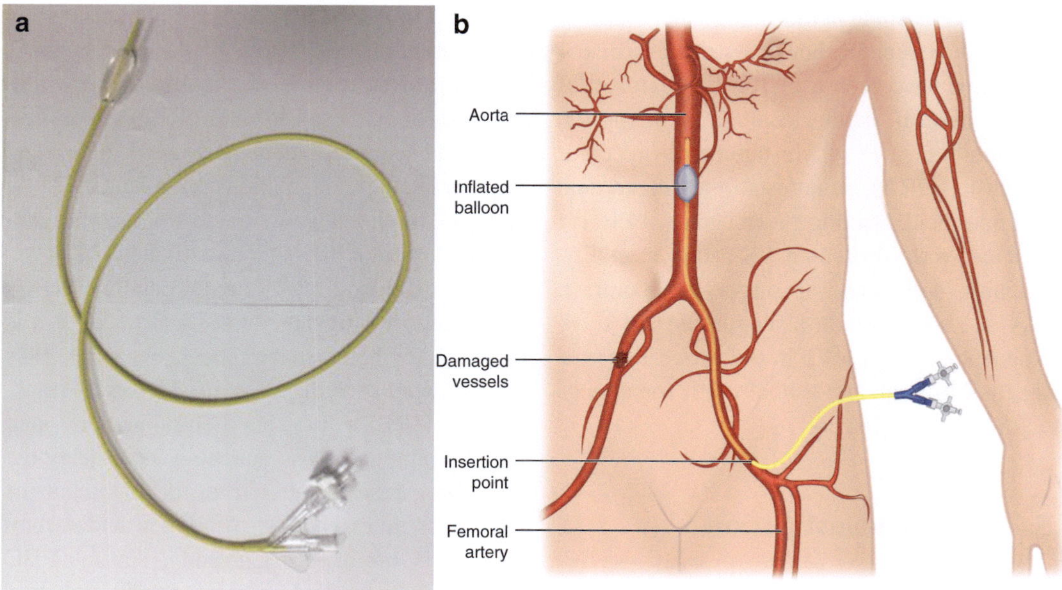

Fig. 2.4 Resuscitative endovascular balloon occlusion of the aorta (REBOA). (**a**) REBOA catheter, (**b**) placement of REBOA

agents include collagen-based, gelatin-based, absorbable cellulose-based agents; fibrin and synthetic glues; and polysaccharide-based agents. These agents are widely used in the traumatic shock currently.

2.4.7.5 Endoscopic Hemostasis and Interventional Approach

Endoscopic hemostasis should be considered in gastrointestinal hemorrhage. Various techniques such as clipping, ligation, and sclerotherapy and drugs such as epinephrine are currently used. In the variceal hemorrhage, balloon tamponade is used as a temporary treatment, and interventional approaches such as trans-jugular intrahepatic portosystemic shunt (TIPS) and balloon-occluded retrograde transvenous obliteration (BRTO) are effective in controlling bleeding and improving prognosis.

2.4.7.6 Pharmacologic Agents for Gastrointestinal Hemorrhage

Upper gastrointestinal hemorrhage is a serious medical condition and it sometimes induces hemorrhagic shock. General management of the upper gastrointestinal hemorrhage is not different with that of traumatic shock. Several pharmacologic agents have been used for the treatment of the non-variceal hemorrhage such as proton pump inhibitors (PPIs), histamine H_2 receptor antagonist (H2RA), somatostatin analogue, and tranexamic acid. Among these agents, PPIs are associated with decreased all-cause mortality, rebleeding, and need for surgery. In contrast, H2RA and somatostatin analogue did not show any beneficial effect [67]. In the variceal hemorrhage, terlipressin and somatostatin analogues are currently used [68].

2.5 Future Investigation

Advances in knowledge regarding the pathophysiology of hemorrhagic shock and many technologies are guiding further investigation.

Prompt control of bleeding is essential in hemorrhagic shock, and coagulation system plays an important role in hemostasis. Recent studies have emphasized on the early administration of plasma, platelets, and coagulation factors and higher ratios of these components to RBC. However, this approach may not be able to provide sufficient supply of the components. Therefore, further investigation of the optimal ratio of plasma and/or platelet to RBC is warranted. Recently, the use of the rapid POCT of coagulation monitoring is increasing, and this could guide the administration of selected clotting factors without considering the fixed ratio. In addition, with the advances in technology, isolated clotting factors and recombinant clotting factors would be easily available, and the results of coagulation system would be taken within minutes.

Donated blood is divided into its separate components and stored because of their various half-lives, but recent massive transfusion protocol includes early administration of coagulation components and often mimics the whole blood transfusion. Alternative methods for the current blood component storage and transfusion are under investigation. Cryopreservation of RBC and platelets has been explored and is currently used in a military [70]. Freeze-dried plasma is a temperature-stable powder and it can be reconstituted with sterile water and administered within minutes. It was used instead of FFP in several European countries and it showed ease of use and improvement of coagulation components [71]. In addition, modified whole blood storage with leukocyte depletion has been investigated [72, 73].

Artificial blood substitutes especially of RBCs have been investigated. Transfusion of RBCs is essential for hemorrhagic shock because RBCs have oxygen-carrying capacity. However, transfusion of RBCs may have complications, and blood typing and cross-matching often delay the rapid transfusion. Therefore, development of RBC substitutes capable of oxygen and carbon dioxide is promising. Currently, several RBC substitutes are studied and they are of mainly two types of perfluorocarbon and hemoglobin-based substitutes [74]. More recently, production of RBCs in laboratory from stems cells is also investigated [75, 76].

In hemorrhagic shock, dysregulated immune responses occur and various anti-inflammatory agents, antioxidants, and immune-modulating agents have been investigated. In addition, hemorrhagic shock may induce the changes of host DNA expression and DNS-modulating agents are also under investigation [77].

Besides blood components and pharmacological agent, another approach is the emergency preservation and resuscitation. It consists of profound induced hypothermia up to 1 h and damage control surgery followed by rewarming and reperfusion. The study for the simple technique of vascular access and pharmacological induction of profound hypothermia is ongoing in the preclinical settings [78].

References

1. Vincent JL, De Backer D. Circulatory shock. N Engl J Med. 2013;369(18):1726–34. https://doi.org/10.1056/NEJMra1208943.
2. Norton R, Kobusingye O. Injuries. N Engl J Med. 2013;368(18):1723–30. https://doi.org/10.1056/NEJMra1109343.
3. Moore K. The physiological response to hemorrhagic shock. J Emerg Nurs. 2014;40(6):629–31. https://doi.org/10.1016/j.jen.2014.08.014.
4. Lord JM, Midwinter MJ, Chen YF, Belli A, Brohi K, Kovacs EJ, et al. The systemic immune response to trauma: an overview of pathophysiology and treatment. Lancet. 2014;384(9952):1455–65. https://doi.org/10.1016/S0140-6736(14)60687-5.
5. Soreide K. Clinical and translational aspects of hypothermia in major trauma patients: from pathophysiology to prevention, prognosis and potential preservation. Injury. 2014;45(4):647–54. https://doi.org/10.1016/j.injury.2012.12.027.
6. Martini WZ, Holcomb JB. Acidosis and coagulopathy: the differential effects on fibrinogen synthesis and breakdown in pigs. Ann Surg. 2007;246(5):831–5. https://doi.org/10.1097/SLA.0b013e3180cc2e94.
7. Wolberg AS, Meng ZH, Monroe DM 3rd, Hoffman M. A systematic evaluation of the effect of temperature on coagulation enzyme activity and platelet function. J Trauma. 2004;56(6):1221–8.
8. Giordano S, Spiezia L, Campello E, Simioni P. The current understanding of trauma-induced coagulopathy (TIC): a focused review on pathophysiology. Intern Emerg Med. 2017; https://doi.org/10.1007/s11739-017-1674-0.
9. Subcommittee A, American College of Surgeons' Committee on T, International Awg. Advanced trauma life support (ATLS(R)): the ninth edition. J Trauma Acute Care Surg. 2013;74(5):1363–6. https://doi.org/10.1097/TA.0b013e31828b82f5.
10. Maegele M. Frequency, risk stratification and therapeutic management of acute post-traumatic coagulopathy. Vox Sang. 2009;97(1):39–49. https://doi.org/10.1111/j.1423-0410.2009.01179.x.
11. Rossaint R, Bouillon B, Cerny V, Coats TJ, Duranteau J, Fernandez-Mondejar E, et al. The European guideline on management of major bleeding and coagulopathy following trauma: fourth edition. Crit Care. 2016;20:100. https://doi.org/10.1186/s13054-016-1265-x.
12. Fox JC, Boysen M, Gharahbaghian L, Cusick S, Ahmed SS, Anderson CL, et al. Test characteristics of focused assessment of sonography for trauma for clinically significant abdominal free fluid in pediatric blunt abdominal trauma. Acad Emerg Med. 2011;18(5):477–82. https://doi.org/10.1111/j.1553-2712.2011.01071.x.
13. Richards JR, Schleper NH, Woo BD, Bohnen PA, McGahan JP. Sonographic assessment of blunt abdominal trauma: a 4-year prospective study. J Clin Ultrasound. 2002;30(2):59–67.
14. Stengel D, Bauwens K, Sehouli J, Porzsolt F, Rademacher G, Mutze S, et al. Systematic review and meta-analysis of emergency ultrasonography for blunt abdominal trauma. Br J Surg. 2001;88(7):901–12. https://doi.org/10.1046/j.0007-1323.2001.01777.x.
15. Becker CD, Poletti PA. The trauma concept: the role of MDCT in the diagnosis and management of visceral injuries. Eur Radiol. 2005;15(Suppl 4):D105–9.
16. Weninger P, Mauritz W, Fridrich P, Spitaler R, Figl M, Kern B, et al. Emergency room management of patients with blunt major trauma: evaluation of the multislice computed tomography protocol exemplified by an urban trauma center. J Trauma. 2007;62(3):584–91. https://doi.org/10.1097/01.ta.0000221797.46249.ee.
17. Anderson SW, Varghese JC, Lucey BC, Burke PA, Hirsch EF, Soto JA. Blunt splenic trauma: delayed-phase CT for differentiation of active hemorrhage from contained vascular injury in patients. Radiology. 2007;243(1):88–95. https://doi.org/10.1148/radiol.2431060376.
18. Wu CH, Wang LJ, Wong YC, Fang JF, Lin BC, Chen HW, et al. Contrast-enhanced multiphasic computed tomography for identifying life-threatening mesenteric hemorrhage and transmural bowel injuries. J Trauma. 2011;71(3):543–8. https://doi.org/10.1097/TA.0b013e3181fef15e.
19. Abramson D, Scalea TM, Hitchcock R, Trooskin SZ, Henry SM, Greenspan J. Lactate clearance and survival following injury. J Trauma. 1993;35(4):584–8; discussion 8–9.
20. Manikis P, Jankowski S, Zhang H, Kahn RJ, Vincent JL. Correlation of serial blood lactate levels to organ failure and mortality after trauma. Am J Emerg Med. 1995;13(6):619–22. https://doi.org/10.1016/0735-6757(95)90043-8.
21. Arnold TD, Miller M, van Wessem KP, Evans JA, Balogh ZJ. Base deficit from the first peripheral venous sample: a surrogate for arterial base defi-

cit in the trauma bay. J Trauma. 2011;71(4):793–7. https://doi.org/10.1097/TA.0b013e31822ad694; discussion 7.
22. Davis JW, Kaups KL, Parks SN. Base deficit is superior to pH in evaluating clearance of acidosis after traumatic shock. J Trauma. 1998;44(1):114–8.
23. MacLeod JB, Lynn M, McKenney MG, Cohn SM, Murtha M. Early coagulopathy predicts mortality in trauma. J Trauma. 2003;55(1):39–44. https://doi.org/10.1097/01.TA.0000075338.21177.EF.
24. Mann KG, Butenas S, Brummel K. The dynamics of thrombin formation. Arterioscler Thromb Vasc Biol. 2003;23(1):17–25.
25. Benes J, Zatloukal J, Kletecka J. Viscoelastic methods of blood clotting assessment—a multidisciplinary review. Front Med. 2015;2:62. https://doi.org/10.3389/fmed.2015.00062.
26. Hanke AA, Horstmann H, Wilhelmi M. Point-of-care monitoring for the management of trauma-induced bleeding. Curr Opin Anaesthesiol. 2017;30(2):250–6. https://doi.org/10.1097/ACO.0000000000000448.
27. Da Luz LT, Nascimento B, Shankarakutty AK, Rizoli S, Adhikari NK. Effect of thromboelastography (TEG(R)) and rotational thromboelastometry (ROTEM(R)) on diagnosis of coagulopathy, transfusion guidance and mortality in trauma: descriptive systematic review. Crit Care. 2014;18(5):518. https://doi.org/10.1186/s13054-014-0518-9.
28. Gonzalez E, Moore EE, Moore HB, Chapman MP, Chin TL, Ghasabyan A, et al. Goal-directed hemostatic resuscitation of trauma-induced coagulopathy: a pragmatic randomized clinical trial comparing a viscoelastic assay to conventional coagulation assays. Ann Surg. 2016;263(6):1051–9. https://doi.org/10.1097/SLA.0000000000001608.
29. Hess JR, Holcomb JB, Hoyt DB. Damage control resuscitation: the need for specific blood products to treat the coagulopathy of trauma. Transfusion. 2006;46(5):685–6. https://doi.org/10.1111/j.1537-2995.2006.00816.x.
30. Briggs A, Askari R. Damage control resuscitation. Int J Surg. 2016;33(Pt B):218–21. https://doi.org/10.1016/j.ijsu.2016.03.064.
31. Camazine MN, Hemmila MR, Leonard JC, Jacobs RA, Horst JA, Kozar RA, et al. Massive transfusion policies at trauma centers participating in the American College of Surgeons Trauma Quality Improvement Program. J Trauma Acute Care Surg. 2015;78(6 Suppl 1):S48–53. https://doi.org/10.1097/TA.0000000000000641.
32. Waydhas C. German Society of Trauma S. [Preclinical management of multiples injuries: S3 guideline]. Unfallchirurg. 2012;115(1):8–13. https://doi.org/10.1007/s00113-011-2102-y.
33. Haut ER, Kalish BT, Cotton BA, Efron DT, Haider AH, Stevens KA, et al. Prehospital intravenous fluid administration is associated with higher mortality in trauma patients: a National Trauma Data Bank analysis. Ann Surg. 2011;253(2):371–7. https://doi.org/10.1097/SLA.0b013e318207c24f.
34. Morrison CA, Carrick MM, Norman MA, Scott BG, Welsh FJ, Tsai P, et al. Hypotensive resuscitation strategy reduces transfusion requirements and severe postoperative coagulopathy in trauma patients with hemorrhagic shock: preliminary results of a randomized controlled trial. J Trauma. 2011;70(3):652–63. https://doi.org/10.1097/TA.0b013e31820e77ea.
35. Berry C, Ley EJ, Bukur M, Malinoski D, Margulies DR, Mirocha J, et al. Redefining hypotension in traumatic brain injury. Injury. 2012;43(11):1833–7. https://doi.org/10.1016/j.injury.2011.08.014.
36. James MF, Michell WL, Joubert IA, Nicol AJ, Navsaria PH, Gillespie RS. Resuscitation with hydroxyethyl starch improves renal function and lactate clearance in penetrating trauma in a randomized controlled study: the FIRST trial (Fluids in Resuscitation of Severe Trauma). Br J Anaesth. 2011;107(5):693–702. https://doi.org/10.1093/bja/aer229.
37. Rasmussen KC, Johansson PI, Hojskov M, Kridina I, Kistorp T, Thind P, et al. Hydroxyethyl starch reduces coagulation competence and increases blood loss during major surgery: results from a randomized controlled trial. Ann Surg. 2014;259(2):249–54. https://doi.org/10.1097/SLA.0000000000000267.
38. Finfer S, Bellomo R, Boyce N, French J, Myburgh J, Norton R, et al. A comparison of albumin and saline for fluid resuscitation in the intensive care unit. N Engl J Med. 2004;350(22):2247–56. https://doi.org/10.1056/NEJMoa040232.
39. Investigators SS, Australian, New Zealand Intensive Care Society Clinical Trials G, Australian Red Cross Blood S, George Institute for International H, Myburgh J et al. Saline or albumin for fluid resuscitation in patients with traumatic brain injury. N Engl J Med. 2007;357(9):874–84. https://doi.org/10.1056/NEJMoa067514.
40. Perel P, Roberts I, Ker K. Colloids versus crystalloids for fluid resuscitation in critically ill patients. Cochrane Database Syst Rev. 2013;2:CD000567. https://doi.org/10.1002/14651858.CD000567.pub6.
41. Yunos NM, Bellomo R, Hegarty C, Story D, Ho L, Bailey M. Association between a chloride-liberal vs chloride-restrictive intravenous fluid administration strategy and kidney injury in critically ill adults. JAMA. 2012;308(15):1566–72. https://doi.org/10.1001/jama.2012.13356.
42. Young JB, Utter GH, Schermer CR, Galante JM, Phan HH, Yang Y, et al. Saline versus Plasma-Lyte A in initial resuscitation of trauma patients: a randomized trial. Ann Surg. 2014;259(2):255–62. https://doi.org/10.1097/SLA.0b013e318295feba.
43. Wade CE, Grady JJ, Kramer GC. Efficacy of hypertonic saline dextran fluid resuscitation for patients with hypotension from penetrating trauma. J Trauma. 2003;54(5 Suppl):S144–8. https://doi.org/10.1097/01.TA.0000047223.62617.AB.
44. Bulger EM, May S, Kerby JD, Emerson S, Stiell IG, Schreiber MA, et al. Out-of-hospital hypertonic resuscitation after traumatic hypovolemic shock: a randomized, placebo controlled trial. Ann

Surg. 2011;253(3):431–41. https://doi.org/10.1097/SLA.0b013e3181fcdb22.
45. Gelman S, Mushlin PS. Catecholamine-induced changes in the splanchnic circulation affecting systemic hemodynamics. Anesthesiology. 2004;100(2):434–9.
46. Kutcher ME, Howard BM, Sperry JL, Hubbard AE, Decker AL, Cuschieri J, et al. Evolving beyond the vicious triad: Differential mediation of traumatic coagulopathy by injury, shock, and resuscitation. J Trauma Acute Care Surg. 2015;78(3):516–23. https://doi.org/10.1097/TA.0000000000000545.
47. Watts DD, Trask A, Soeken K, Perdue P, Dols S, Kaufmann C. Hypothermic coagulopathy in trauma: effect of varying levels of hypothermia on enzyme speed, platelet function, and fibrinolytic activity. J Trauma. 1998;44(5):846–54.
48. Bernabei AF, Levison MA, Bender JS. The effects of hypothermia and injury severity on blood loss during trauma laparotomy. J Trauma. 1992;33(6):835–9.
49. Hoey BA, Schwab CW. Damage control surgery. Scand J Surg. 2002;91(1):92–103. https://doi.org/10.1177/145749690209100115.
50. Holcomb JB, Donathan DP, Cotton BA, Del Junco DJ, Brown G, Wenckstern TV, et al. Prehospital transfusion of plasma and red blood cells in trauma patients. Prehosp Emerg Care. 2015a;19(1):1–9. https://doi.org/10.3109/10903127.2014.923077.
51. Rahbar E, Fox EE, del Junco DJ, Harvin JA, Holcomb JB, Wade CE, et al. Early resuscitation intensity as a surrogate for bleeding severity and early mortality in the PROMMTT study. J Trauma Acute Care Surg. 2013;75(1 Suppl 1):S16–23. https://doi.org/10.1097/TA.0b013e31828fa535.
52. Savage SA, Zarzaur BL, Croce MA, Fabian TC. Redefining massive transfusion when every second counts. J Trauma Acute Care Surg. 2013;74(2):396–400. https://doi.org/10.1097/TA.0b013e31827a3639; discussion -2.
53. Cantle PM, Cotton BA. Prediction of massive transfusion in trauma. Crit Care Clin. 2017;33(1):71–84. https://doi.org/10.1016/j.ccc.2016.08.002.
54. Nunez TC, Voskresensky IV, Dossett LA, Shinall R, Dutton WD, Cotton BA. Early prediction of massive transfusion in trauma: simple as ABC (assessment of blood consumption)? J Trauma. 2009;66(2):346–52. https://doi.org/10.1097/TA.0b013e3181961c35.
55. Dente CJ, Shaz BH, Nicholas JM, Harris RS, Wyrzykowski AD, Patel S, et al. Improvements in early mortality and coagulopathy are sustained better in patients with blunt trauma after institution of a massive transfusion protocol in a civilian level I trauma center. J Trauma. 2009;66(6):1616–24. https://doi.org/10.1097/TA.0b013e3181a59ad5.
56. Savage SA, Zarzaur BL, Croce MA, Fabian TC. Time matters in 1: 1 resuscitations: concurrent administration of blood: plasma and risk of death. J Trauma Acute Care Surg. 2014;77(6):833–7. https://doi.org/10.1097/TA.0000000000000355; discussion 7–8.
57. Holcomb JB, del Junco DJ, Fox EE, Wade CE, Cohen MJ, Schreiber MA, et al. The prospective, observational, multicenter, major trauma transfusion (PROMMTT) study: comparative effectiveness of a time-varying treatment with competing risks. JAMA Surg. 2013;148(2):127–36. https://doi.org/10.1001/2013.jamasurg.387.
58. Ho AM, Dion PW, Yeung JH, Holcomb JB, Critchley LA, Ng CS, et al. Prevalence of survivor bias in observational studies on fresh frozen plasma: erythrocyte ratios in trauma requiring massive transfusion. Anesthesiology. 2012;116(3):716–28. https://doi.org/10.1097/ALN.0b013e318245c47b.
59. Holcomb JB, Tilley BC, Baraniuk S, Fox EE, Wade CE, Podbielski JM, et al. Transfusion of plasma, platelets, and red blood cells in a 1:1:1 vs a 1:1:2 ratio and mortality in patients with severe trauma: the PROPPR randomized clinical trial. JAMA. 2015b;313(5):471–82. https://doi.org/10.1001/jama.2015.12.
60. Stinger HK, Spinella PC, Perkins JG, Grathwohl KW, Salinas J, Martini WZ, et al. The ratio of fibrinogen to red cells transfused affects survival in casualties receiving massive transfusions at an army combat support hospital. J Trauma. 2008;64(2 Suppl):S79–85. https://doi.org/10.1097/TA.0b013e318160a57b; discussion S.
61. Cole E, Davenport R, Willett K, Brohi K. Tranexamic acid use in severely injured civilian patients and the effects on outcomes: a prospective cohort study. Ann Surg. 2015;261(2):390–4. https://doi.org/10.1097/SLA.0000000000000717.
62. Collaborators C, Shakur H, Roberts I, Bautista R, Caballero J, Coats T, et al. Effects of tranexamic acid on death, vascular occlusive events, and blood transfusion in trauma patients with significant haemorrhage (CRASH-2): a randomised, placebo-controlled trial. Lancet. 2010;376(9734):23–32. https://doi.org/10.1016/S0140-6736(10)60835-5.
63. Collaborators C, Roberts I, Shakur H, Afolabi A, Brohi K, Coats T, et al. The importance of early treatment with tranexamic acid in bleeding trauma patients: an exploratory analysis of the CRASH-2 randomised controlled trial. Lancet. 2011;377(9771):1096–101, 101 e1–2. https://doi.org/10.1016/S0140-6736(11)60278-X.
64. Collaborators WT. Effect of early tranexamic acid administration on mortality, hysterectomy, and other morbidities in women with post-partum haemorrhage (WOMAN): an international, randomised, double-blind, placebo-controlled trial. Lancet. 2017;389(10084):2105–16. https://doi.org/10.1016/S0140-6736(17)30638-4.
65. Ho KM, Leonard AD. Concentration-dependent effect of hypocalcaemia on mortality of patients with critical bleeding requiring massive transfusion: a cohort study. Anaesth Intensive Care. 2011;39(1):46–54.
66. Magnotti LJ, Bradburn EH, Webb DL, Berry SD, Fischer PE, Zarzaur BL, et al. Admission ionized calcium levels predict the need for multiple transfusions: a prospective study of 591 critically ill trauma

patients. J Trauma. 2011;70(2):391–5. https://doi.org/10.1097/TA.0b013e31820b5d98; discussion 5–7.
67. Jiang M, Chen P, Gao Q. Systematic review and net-work meta-analysis of upper gastrointestinal hemorrhage interventions. Cell Physiol Biochem. 2016;39(6):2477–91. https://doi.org/10.1159/000452515.
68. Hernandez-Gea V, Berbel C, Baiges A, Garcia-Pagan JC. Acute variceal bleeding: risk stratification and management (including TIPS). Hepatol Int. 2017; https://doi.org/10.1007/s12072-017-9804-3.
69. Morrison JJ, Galgon RE, Jansen JO, Cannon JW, Rasmussen TE, Eliason JL. A systematic review of the use of resuscitative endovascular balloon occlusion of the aorta in the management of hemorrhagic shock. J Trauma Acute Care Surg. 2016;80(2):324–34. https://doi.org/10.1097/TA.0000000000000913.
70. Lelkens CC, Koning JG, de Kort B, Floot IB, Noorman F. Experiences with frozen blood products in the Netherlands military. Transfus Apher Sci. 2006;34(3):289–98. https://doi.org/10.1016/j.transci.2005.11.008.
71. Martinaud C, Ausset S, Deshayes AV, Cauet A, Demazeau N, Sailliol A. Use of freeze-dried plasma in French intensive care unit in Afghanistan. J Trauma. 2011;71(6):1761–4. https://doi.org/10.1097/TA.0b013e31822f1285; discussion 4–5.
72. Murdock AD, Berseus O, Hervig T, Strandenes G, Lunde TH. Whole blood: the future of traumatic hemorrhagic shock resuscitation. Shock. 2014;41(Suppl 1):62–9. https://doi.org/10.1097/SHK.0000000000000134.
73. Snyder EL, Whitley P, Kingsbury T, Miripol J, Tormey CA. In vitro and in vivo evaluation of a whole blood platelet-sparing leukoreduction filtration system. Transfusion. 2010;50(10):2145–51. https://doi.org/10.1111/j.1537-2995.2010.02701.x.
74. Moradi S, Jahanian-Najafabadi A, Roudkenar MH. Artificial blood substitutes: first steps on the long route to clinical utility. Clin Med Insights Blood Disord. 2016;9:33–41. https://doi.org/10.4137/CMBD.S38461.
75. Hirose S, Takayama N, Nakamura S, Nagasawa K, Ochi K, Hirata S, et al. Immortalization of erythroblasts by c-MYC and BCL-XL enables large-scale erythrocyte production from human pluripotent stem cells. Stem Cell Rep. 2013;1(6):499–508. https://doi.org/10.1016/j.stemcr.2013.10.010.
76. Olivier E, Qiu C, Bouhassira EE. Novel, high-yield red blood cell production methods from CD34-positive cells derived from human embryonic stem, yolk sac, fetal liver, cord blood, and peripheral blood. Stem Cells Transl Med. 2012;1(8):604–14. https://doi.org/10.5966/sctm.2012-0059.
77. Martin DT, Schreiber MA. Modern resuscitation of hemorrhagic shock: what is on the horizon? Eur J Trauma Emerg Surg. 2014;40(6):641–56. https://doi.org/10.1007/s00068-014-0416-5.
78. Kutcher ME, Forsythe RM, Tisherman SA. Emergency preservation and resuscitation for cardiac arrest from trauma. Int J Surg. 2016;33(Pt B):209–12. https://doi.org/10.1016/j.ijsu.2015.10.014.

3 Cardiogenic Shock

Jonghwan Shin

3.1 Introduction

Cardiogenic shock is a serious complication of acute myocardial infarction and is an important cause of hospital death. Cardiogenic shock is a condition in which your heart suddenly can't pump enough blood to meet your body's needs. The condition is most often caused by a severe heart attack. Cardiogenic shock is rare, but it's often fatal if not treated immediately. If treated immediately, about half the people who develop the condition survive. The incidence of cardiogenic shock is about 5% in patients with acute myocardial infarction (AMI) and three times more ST-segment elevation myocardial infarction (STEMI) than in non-STEMI [1]. Recent advances in early treatment, technological advancement, and pharmacologic treatment have improved the prognosis of patients and improved long-term survival and quality of life. Therefore, the mortality rate due to cardiogenic shock is also decreasing, and the prognosis of the high-risk patients is better than the previous one [2].

Table 3.1 The definition of CS consists of hemodynamic instability of various parameters

I.	Persistent hypotension: systolic blood pressure <90 mmHg or mean arterial pressure 30 mmHg lower than baseline
II.	Severe reduction in cardiac index: <1.8 L/min/m^2 without support or <2.0–2.2 L/min/m^2 with support
III.	Adequate or elevated filling pressure: left ventricular end-diastolic pressure >18 mmHg or right ventricular end-diastolic pressure >10–15 mmHg.

3.2 Definition of Cardiogenic Shock

Cardiogenic shock is a life-threatening medical condition resulting from an inadequate circulation of blood due to primary failure of the ventricles of the heart to function effectively (Table 3.1). Signs of tissue hypoperfusion include low urine production, cool extremities, and altered mental of consciousness.

3.3 Pathophysiology

The most common cause of cardiogenic shock is pump failure due to extensive myocardial infarction (MI) with damage to the heart muscle and subsequent depression of myocardial contractility. Additional causes of cardiogenic shock are listed in Table 3.2 [3]. Other mechanical

J. Shin
Department of Emergency Medicine, Seoul National University College of Medicine,
Seoul, South Korea

G. J. Suh (ed.), *Essentials of Shock Management*, https://doi.org/10.1007/978-981-10-5406-8_3

Table 3.2 Causes of cardiogenic shock

Acute myocardial infarction
Pump failure
Large infarction
Smaller infarction with preexisting left ventricular dysfunction
Infarction extension
Reinfarction
Infarction expansion
Mechanical complications
Acute mitral regurgitation caused by papillary muscle rupture
Ventricular septal defect
Free-wall rupture
Pericardial tamponade
Right ventricular infarction
Other conditions
End-stage cardiomyopathy
Myocarditis
Myocardial contusion
Prolonged cardiopulmonary bypass
Septic shock with severe myocardial depression
Left ventricular outflow tract obstruction
Aortic stenosis
Hypertrophic obstructive cardiomyopathy
Obstruction to left ventricular filing
Mitral stenosis
Left atrial myxoma
Acute mitral regurgitation (chordal rupture)
Acute aortic insufficiency

complications following myocardial injury after MI are acute mitral regurgitation resulting from papillary muscle rupture, ventricular septal defect, and free-wall rupture. Mechanical complication must be strongly suspected in patients with cardiogenic shock complicating non-anterior MI, especially complications of a first MI.

Sepsis, hemorrhage, and bowel ischemia also cause cardiogenic shock, which severely reduces the myocardial contractility. These causes require proper treatment through suspicion or recognition of the cause as well as support of the myocardial function.

Acute myocarditis, takotsubo cardiomyopathy, hypertrophic cardiomyopathy, and myocardial contusion may lead to cardiogenic shock in the absence of significant coronary artery disease. Acute valvular regurgitation of left ventricular (LV) output caused by endocarditis or chordal rupture may also cause cardiogenic shock. Acute aortic insufficiency due to aortic dissection, cardiac tamponade, or massive pulmonary embolism can present as cardiogenic shock without associated pulmonary edema.

Cardiogenic shock is a clinical syndrome characterized by systemic hypotension and hypoperfusion secondary to insufficient cardiac output. LV pump failure is a major cause of cardiogenic shock, but right ventricular (RV) failure and macro/microcirculation system are also responsible for cardiogenic shock. Recent research has suggested that the peripheral vasculature, neurohormonal, and cytokine systems play a role in the pathogenesis and persistence of cardiogenic shock [4–10].

In general, myocardial dysfunction is severe enough to cause cardiogenic shock. In the case of cardiogenic shock, myocardial contractility disturbance causes a decrease in the afterload, lowering the blood pressure, resulting in systemic hypoperfusion. The mean depression of LV ejection fraction (EF) is moderate to severe (30%), with a wide range of EF and LV sizes recorded [11]. Metabolic disorders occur in the areas of the remote myocardium and in the infarct region [12]. Hypoperfusion causes release of catecholamines, which increase contractility and peripheral blood flow, but catecholamines also increase myocardial oxygen demand and cause proarrhythmic and myocardiotoxic effects. Cardiogenic shock is not the only result of severe depression of LV function due to extensive myocardial ischemia or injury. Depressed myocardial contractility is accompanied by inadequate systemic vasoconstriction as a result from a systemic inflammatory response to extensive myocardial injury in cardiogenic shock.

RV failure can contribute to cardiogenic shock, but the ratio of predominant cardiogenic shock due to mainly RV failure is only 5% [13]. However, cardiogenic shock due to isolated RV failure is associated with a higher risk of death, as with LV failure. RV failure reduces cardiac output and ventricular interdependence, eventually decreasing LV filling. Treatment of RV failure with cardiogenic shock is focused on ensuring adequate right-heart filling pressure to maintain cardiac output and adequate LV preload.

Decreased cardiac output due to MI and progressive myocardial ischemia cause the release of catecholamines, which constrict peripheral arterial vessels to maintain the perfusion of important organs. Activation of the neurohormone cascade promotes salt and moisture retention. This can improve perfusion, but worsens pulmonary edema.

The reflex mechanism of increased systemic vascular resistance (SVR) is not generally effective, as evidenced by the variable SVR, with average SVR during cardiogenic shock in the normal range despite vasopressor therapy [14].

Excess nitric oxide (NO) can also contribute to systemic inflammatory response syndrome. MI is associated with increased expression of inducible NO synthase, which leads to excess NO, which inhibits vasoconstriction, myocardial function, and catecholamine action [9, 10].

3.4 Treatment and Management

3.4.1 Initial Approach and Diagnosis

Cardiogenic shock is defined as hypotension (SBP <90 mmHg) despite adequate filling status with signs of hypoperfusion. A patient in cardiogenic shock should undergo immediate comprehensive assessment. Chest X-ray, electrocardiogram (ECG), and echocardiography are required immediately in all patients with suspected cardiogenic shock. Chest X-ray can be a useful test for the diagnosis of cardiogenic shock. Pulmonary venous congestion, pleural effusion, interstitial or alveolar edema, and cardiomegaly are the most specific findings for cardiogenic shock, although in up to 20% of patients with cardiogenic shock chest X-ray is nearly normal [15]. ECG is rarely normal in cardiogenic shock. It is also helpful in identifying underlying cardiac disease and potential precipitants [16]. Immediate echocardiography is mandatory only in patients with hemodynamic instability in cardiogenic shock and in patients suspected of acute life-threatening structural or functional cardiac abnormalities. The following laboratory assessments should be performed at admission on the blood of all patients with cardiogenic shock: cardiac troponin, natriuretic peptides (BNP), blood urea nitrogen (BUN), creatinine, electrolytes (sodium, potassium), liver function tests, thyroid-stimulating hormone (TSH), serum glucose complete blood count, and D-dimer.

A plasma BNP level should be measured in all patients with acute dyspnea and suspected cardiogenic shock to help in the differentiation of cardiogenic shock from noncardiac causes of acute dyspnea. BNP have high sensitivity, and normal levels in patients with suspected acute heart failure make the diagnosis unlikely [17–21]. The level of BNP is an important predictor of cardiovascular events (reinfarction, cardiogenic shock, sustained ventricular tachycardia, ventricular fibrillation, angina, symptoms of left ventricular dysfunction) in patients with acute coronary syndrome and provides better predictive power than the troponin level [22].

Measurement of cardiac troponin is useful for detection of acute coronary syndrome (ACS) as the underlying cause of cardiogenic shock. However, elevated concentrations of circulating cardiac troponins are detected in the vast majority of patients with cardiogenic shock, often without obvious myocardial ischemia or an acute coronary event, suggesting ongoing myocyte injury or necrosis in these patients [23]. The patients of cardiogenic shock have been found to have close association with increased level of serum cardiac troponin-I. The troponin ratio was independently associated with the development of cardiogenic shock [24, 25].

In patients with cardiogenic shock complicating ACS, an immediate coronary angiography is recommended with an intent to perform coronary revascularization. Invasive monitoring with an arterial line should also be considered.

3.4.2 General Support Measures

Prehospital emergency medical service should be considered for transfer to a specialized cardiac care center if cardiogenic shock is suspected. Emergency department care is a temporizing measure during the preparation for revascularization in the cardiac catheterization laboratory or surgical intervention for mechanical failure.

Antithrombotic therapy with aspirin and heparin should be given as routinely recommended for MI. Clopidogrel may be deferred until after emergency angiography, because on the basis of angiographic findings coronary artery bypass grafting (CABG) may be performed immediately. Clopidogrel is indicated in all patients who undergo percutaneous coronary intervention (PCI), and on the basis of extrapolation of data from MI patients who were not in shock it should also be useful in patients with shock as well. Negative inotropes and vasodilators (including nitroglycerin) should be avoided. Arterial oxygenation and near-normal pH should be maintained to minimize ischemia. Intensive insulin therapy improves survival in hyperglycemic critically ill patients and is recommended for use in complicated MI. There should be a low threshold to institute mechanical ventilation via mask or endotracheal tube. Positive end-expiratory pressure decreases preload and afterload. Mechanical ventilation also reduces work of breathing (Fig. 3.1).

3.4.3 Hemodynamic Management

Fluid is given in RV infarct with hypotension. Because some patients with cardiogenic shock develop hypotension without pulmonary edema, an appropriate amount of fluid can be administered. If there is no improvement in perfusion with fluid challenge, or there is hypoperfusion with pulmonary edema, vasopressors or inotropes are considered.

Pulmonary artery (PA) catheterization is frequently performed to confirm the diagnosis of cardiogenic shock, to ensure adequate filling pressure, and to guide changes in therapy. Individualized PA catheter use is recommended for MI patients with severe hypotension [26]. However, many centers have chosen to manage cardiogenic shock without PA catheterization. Clinical evaluation with echocardiography is a reasonable alternative. Both PA systolic pressure and wedge pressure can be accurately estimated with Doppler echocardiography, and in particular the finding of a short mitral deceleration time

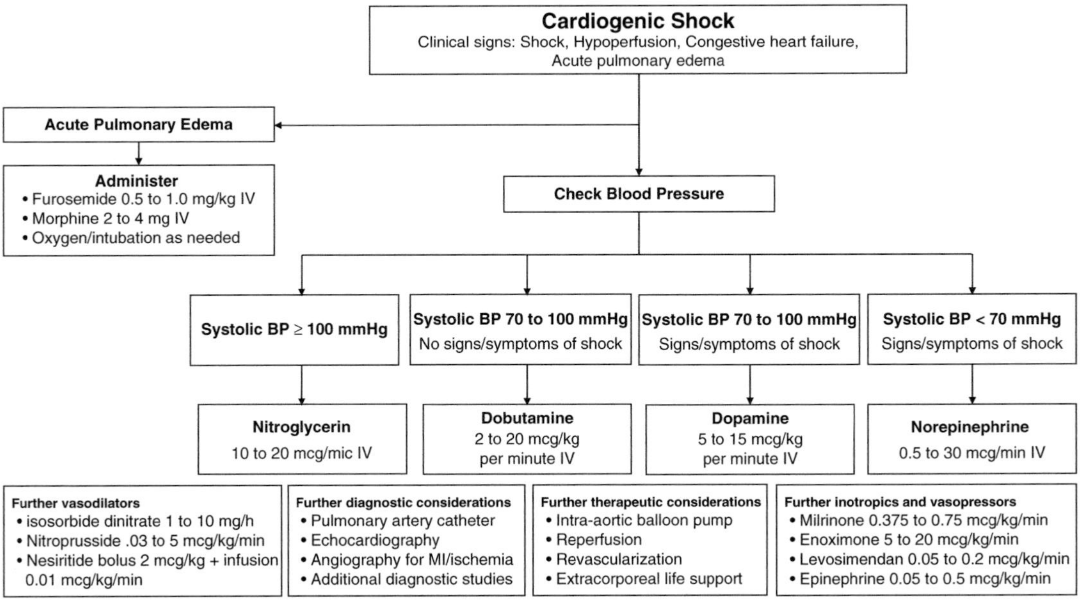

Fig. 3.1 Emergency management of complicated ST-elevation myocardial infarction. The emergency management of patients with cardiogenic shock, acute pulmonary edema, or both is outlined. *SBP* systolic blood pressure, *IV* intravenous, *BP* blood pressure, *MI* myocardial infarction. *Furosemide less than 0.5 mg/kg for new-onset acute pulmonary edema without hypovolemia; 1 mg/kg for acute or chronic volume overload, and renal insufficiency. Combinations of medications, e.g., dobutamine and dopamine, may be used

(≤140 ms) is highly predictive of pulmonary capillary wedge pressure ≥20 mm Hg in cardiogenic shock [27].

Pharmacological treatment, such as inotropic and vasopressor agents, should be used in the lowest possible doses. Higher vasopressor doses are associated with poorer survival [28]. This indicates both severe hemodynamic disturbances and direct toxic effects. Use of inotropic and vasopressor agents is always required to maintain coronary and systemic perfusion until the IABP is placed or until the shock is resolved. There are very little studies on comparisons of vasopressors. The American College of Cardiology/American Heart Association guidelines recommend norepinephrine for more severe hypotension due to its high potency [26]. Although norepinephrine has inotropic properties, dobutamine is often necessary in this condition. Use of dopamine in this setting can be associated with excess risk [29].

Levosimendan may also be used in combination with an inotropic agent or vasopressor. Levosimendan infusion in severe cardiogenic shock complicating AMI in addition to dobutamine and norepinephrine improved survival and cardiovascular hemodynamics without leading to hypotension [30, 31]. Milrinone can also be another alternative to nonischemic patients [32, 33].

3.4.4 Mechanical Support (Fig. 3.2)

Intra-aortic balloon pump (IABP) counterpulsation has long been the mainstay of mechanical therapy for cardiogenic shock. Use of an IABP improves coronary and peripheral perfusion via diastolic balloon inflation and augments LV performance via systolic balloon deflation with an acute decrease in afterload. Accurate timing of inflation and deflation provides optimal support. Not every patient has a hemodynamic response to IABP; response predicts better outcome [34]. IABP support should be instituted as quickly as possible, even before any transfer for revascularization if a skilled operator is available and insertion can be performed quickly.

The use of IABP counterpulsation can be useful for patients with cardiogenic shock after STEMI who do not quickly stabilize with pharmacological therapy [35].

In the large National Registry of Myocardial Infarction, IABP use was independently associated with survival at centers with higher rates of IABP use, whether PCI, fibrinolytic therapy, or no reperfusion had been used [36]. Complications associated with IABP are less common in the modern era; in the largest series, the overall and major complication rates were 7.2% and 2.8%, respectively [37] (Fig. 3.3).

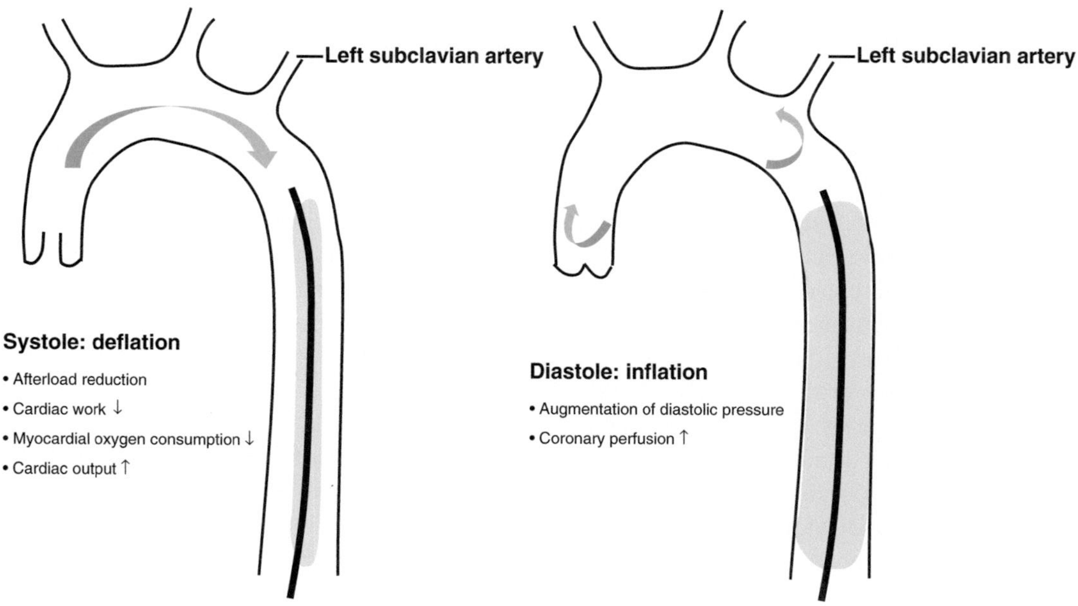

Fig. 3.2 Intra-aortic counterpulsation balloon pump

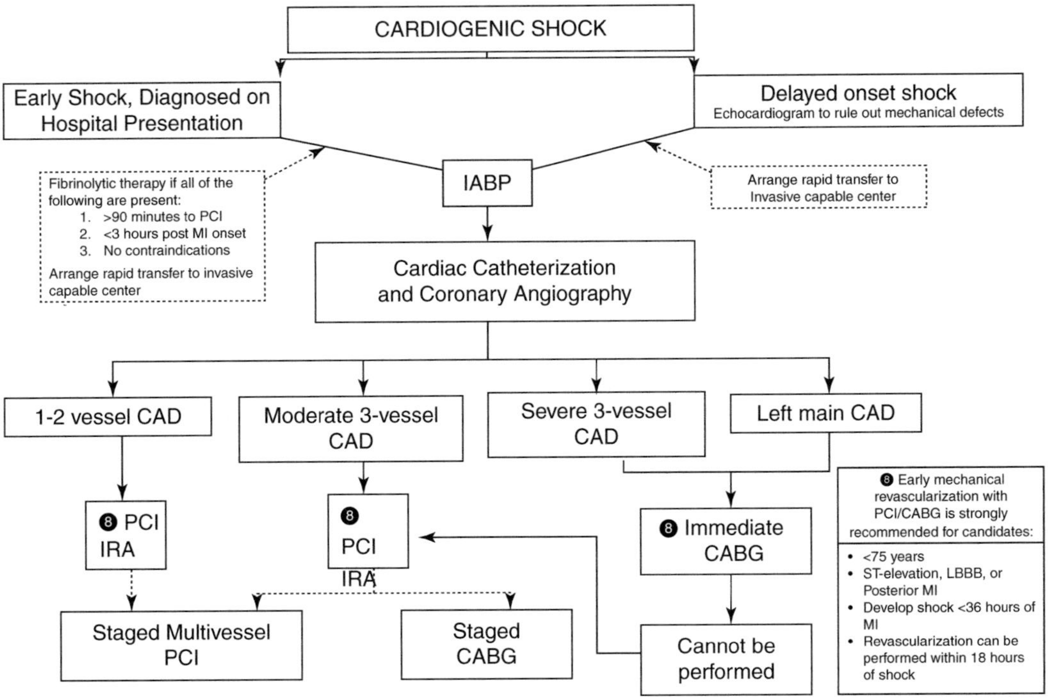

Fig. 3.3 Recommendations for initial reperfusion therapy when cardiogenic shock complicates acute MI. Early mechanical revascularization with PCI or CABG is strongly recommended for suitable candidates 75 years of age and for selected elderly patients (see text). Eighty-five percent of shock cases are diagnosed after initial therapy for acute MI, but most patients develop shock within 24 h. Intra-aortic balloon pump (IABP) is recommended when shock is not quickly reversed with pharmacological therapy, as a stabilizing measure for patients who are candidates for further invasive care. Dashed lines indicate that the procedure should be performed in patients with specific indications only. Recommendations for staged CABG and multivessel PCI are discussed in the text, as are definitions of moderate and severe three-vessel CAD. LBBB indicates left bundle-branch block (*Circulation* 2003;107:2998–3002)

3.4.5 Reperfusion

The survival benefit of early revascularization in cardiogenic shock, reported in several observational studies, was shown convincingly in the randomized SHOCK trial, which found a 13% absolute increase in 1-year survival in patients assigned to early revascularization [11, 38].

Emergency revascularization with either PCI or CABG is recommended in suitable patients with cardiogenic shock due to pump failure after STEMI irrespective of the time delay from MI onset [35]. In the absence of contraindications, fibrinolytic therapy should be administered to patients with STEMI and cardiogenic shock who are unsuitable candidates for either PCI or CABG [31]. Thrombolytic therapy is less effective but is indicated when PCI is impossible or if a delay has occurred in transport for PCI and when MI and cardiogenic shock onset were within 3 h.

As in MI without shock, earlier revascularization is better in cardiogenic shock. Presentation 0–6 h after symptom onset was associated with the lowest mortality among cardiogenic shock patients undergoing primary PCI, in which door-to-angiography times were <90 min in approximately three-fourths of patients [39].

3.4.6 Revascularization Approach: Surgery or PCI (Fig. 3.2)

Revascularization in the SHOCK trial could be percutaneous or surgical. Thirty-seven percent of patients assigned to the early revascularization strategy underwent CABG at a median of 2.7 h after randomization [40]. Despite a higher prevalence of triple-vessel or left main disease and diabetes mellitus in patients who underwent CABG compared with PCI, survival and quality of life were similar [40, 41].

3.4.7 Total Circulatory Support: LV Assist Devices and Extracorporeal Life Support

Temporary mechanical circulatory support with LV assist devices is theoretically appealing to interrupt the vicious spiral of ischemia, hypotension, and myocardial dysfunction, allowing for recovery of stunned and hibernating myocardium and reversal of neurohormonal derangements. Device-related complications and irreversible organ failure remain major limitations.

Compared with IABP, LV assist devices may provide superior hemodynamic support and serve as more effective bridges to recovery or transplantation, though experience with their use in this setting is limited [42, 43].

Alternative LV assist devices for circulatory support may be considered in patients with refractory cardiogenic shock [35] (Fig. 3.4).

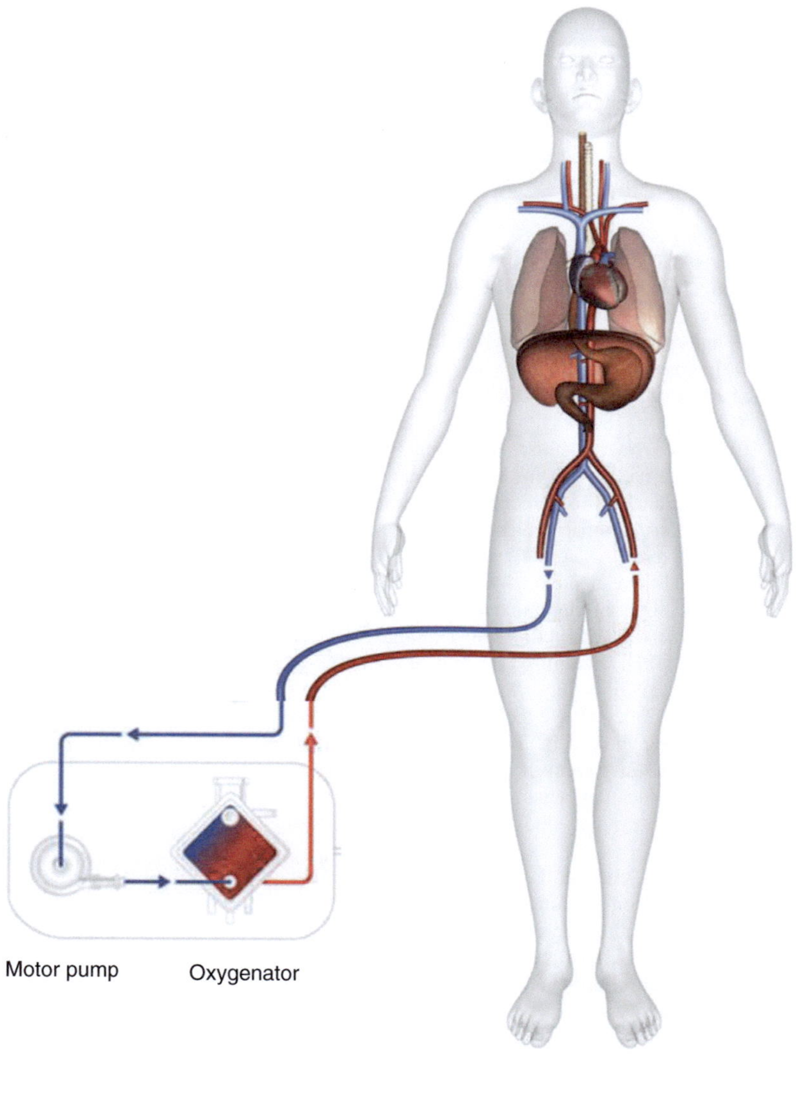

Fig. 3.4 LV assist device and extracorporeal life support

References

1. Nguyen HL, Yarzebski J, Lessard D, et al. Ten-year (2001–2011) trends in the incidence rates and short-term outcomes of early versus late onset cardiogenic shock after hospitalization for acute myocardial infarction. J Am Heart Assoc. 2017;6(6):pii: e005566. https://doi.org/10.1161/JAHA.117.005566.
2. Davierwala PM, Leontyev S, Verevkin A, et al. Temporal trends in predictors of early and late mortality after emergency coronary artery bypass grafting for cardiogenic shock complicating acute myocardial infarction. Circulation. 2016;134(17):1224–37.
3. Hollenberg SM, Kavinsky CJ, Parrillo JE. Cardiogenic shock. Ann Intern Med. 1999;131(1):47–59.
4. Brunkhorst FM, Clark AL, Forycki ZF, et al. Pyrexia, procalcitonin, immune activation and survival in cardiogenic shock: the potential importance of bacterial translocation. Int J Cardiol. 1999;72(1):3–10.
5. Théroux P, Armstrong PW, Mahaffey KW, et al. Prognostic significance of blood markers of inflammation in patients with ST-segment elevation myocardial infarction undergoing primary angioplasty and effects of pexelizumab, a C5 inhibitor: a substudy of the COMMA trial. Eur Heart J. 2005;26(19):1964–70.
6. Zhang C, Xu X, Potter BJ, et al. TNF-alpha contributes to endothelial dysfunction in ischemia/reperfusion injury. Arterioscler Thromb Vasc Biol. 2006;26(3):475–80.
7. Granger CB, Mahaffey KW, Weaver WD, et al. Pexelizumab, an anti-C5 complement antibody, as adjunctive therapy to primary percutaneous coronary intervention in acute myocardial infarction: the COMplement inhibition in Myocardial infarction treated with Angioplasty (COMMA) trial. Circulation. 2003;108(10):1184–90.
8. APEX AMI Investigators, Armstrong PW, Granger CB, et al. Pexelizumab for acute ST-elevation myocardial infarction in patients undergoing primary percutaneous coronary intervention: a randomized controlled trial. JAMA. 2007;297(1):43–51.
9. TRIUMPH Investigators, Alexander JH, Reynolds HR, et al. Effect of tilarginine acetate in patients with acute myocardial infarction and cardiogenic shock: the TRIUMPH randomized controlled trial. JAMA. 2007;297(15):1657–66.
10. Dzavík V, Cotter G, Reynolds HR, et al. Effect of nitric oxide synthase inhibition on haemodynamics and outcome of patients with persistent cardiogenic shock complicating acute myocardial infarction: a phase II dose-ranging study. Eur Heart J. 2007;28(9): 1109–16.
11. Hochman JS, Sleeper LA, Webb JG, et al. Early revascularization in acute myocardial infarction complicated by cardiogenic shock. SHOCK Investigators. Should We Emergently Revascularize Occluded Coronaries for Cardiogenic Shock. N Engl J Med. 1999;341(9):625–34.
12. Beyersdorf F, Buckberg GD, Acar C, et al. Cardiogenic shock after acute coronary occlusion. Pathogenesis, early diagnosis, and treatment. Thorac Cardiovasc Surg. 1989;37(1):28–36.
13. Jacobs AK, Leopold JA, Bates E, et al. Cardiogenic shock caused by right ventricular infarction: a report from the SHOCK registry. J Am Coll Cardiol. 2003;41(8):1273–9.
14. Kohsaka S, Menon V, Lowe AM, et al. Systemic inflammatory response syndrome after acute myocardial infarction complicated by cardiogenic shock. Arch Intern Med. 2005;165(14):1643–50.
15. Chakko S, Woska D, Martinez H, et al. Clinical, radiographic, and hemodynamic correlations in chronic congestive heart failure: conflicting results may lead to inappropriate care. Am J Med. 1991;90(3):353–9.
16. Wang CS, FitzGerald JM, Schulzer M, et al. Does this dyspneic patient in the emergency department have congestive heart failure? JAMA. 2005;294(15):1944–56.
17. Fuat A, Murphy JJ, Hungin AP, et al. The diagnostic accuracy and utility of a B-type natriuretic peptide test in a community population of patients with suspected heart failure. Br J Gen Pract. 2006;56(526):327–33.
18. Yamamoto K, Burnett JC Jr, Bermudez EA, et al. Clinical criteria and biochemical markers for the detection of systolic dysfunction. J Card Fail. 2000;6(3):194–200.
19. Cowie MR, Struthers AD, Wood DA, et al. Value of natriuretic peptides in assessment of patients with possible new heart failure in primary care. Lancet. 1997;350(9088):1349–53.
20. Krishnaswamy P, Lubien E, Clopton P, et al. Utility of B-natriuretic peptide levels in identifying patients with left ventricular systolic or diastolic dysfunction. Am J Med. 2001;111(4):274–9.
21. Kelder JC, Cramer MJ, Verweij WM, et al. Clinical utility of three B-type natriuretic peptide assays for the initial diagnostic assessment of new slow-onset heart failure. J Card Fail. 2011;17(9):729–34.
22. Vogiatzis I, Dapcevic I, Datsios A, et al. A comparison of prognostic value of the levels of ProBNP and troponin T in patients with acute coronary syndrome (ACS). Mediev Archaeol. 2016;70:269–73.
23. Felker GM, Mentz RJ, Teerlink JR, et al. Serial high sensitivity cardiac troponin T measurement in acute heart failure: insights from the RELAX-AHF study. Eur J Heart Fail. 2015;17(12):1262–70.
24. Rukunuzzman M, Latif SA, Rahman M-U, Kirtania K, Islam MT, Ali MO, Hassan MM. Studies on cardiac troponin i in patients with cardiogenic shock. J Dhaka National Med Coll Hos. 2012;18:21–3.
25. Jolly SS, Shenkman H, Brieger D, et al. Quantitative troponin and death, cardiogenic shock, cardiac arrest and new heart failure in patients with non-ST-segment elevation acute coronary syndromes (NSTE ACS): insight from the Global Registry of Acute Coronary Events. Heart. 2011;97(3):197–202.

26. Antman EM, Anbe DT, Armstrong PW, et al. ACC/AHA guidelines for the management of patients with ST-elevation myocardial infarction—executive summary: a report of the American College of Cardiology/American Heart Association Task Force on Practice Guidelines (Writing Committee to Revise the 1999 Guidelines for the Management of Patients With Acute Myocardial Infarction). Circulation. 2004;110(5):588–636.
27. Reynolds HR, Anand SK, Fox JM, et al. Restrictive physiology in cardiogenic shock: observations from echocardiography. Am Heart J. 2006;151:890.e9–e15.
28. Valente S, Lazzeri C, Vecchio S, et al. Predictors of in-hospital mortality after percutaneous coronary intervention for cardiogenic shock. Int J Cardiol. 2007;114(2):176–82.
29. De Backer D, Biston P, Devriendt J, et al. Comparison of dopamine and norepinephrine in the treatment of shock. N Engl J Med. 2010;362(9):779–89.
30. Russ MA, Prondzinsky R, Christoph A, et al. Hemodynamic improvement following levosimendan treatment in patients with acute myocardial infarction and cardiogenic shock. Crit Care Med. 2007;35:2732–9.
31. Fuhrmann JT, Schmeisser A, Schulze MR, et al. Levosimendan is superior to enoximone in refractory cardiogenic shock complicating acute myocardial infarction. Crit Care Med. 2008;36:2257–66.
32. Cuffe MS, Califf RM, Adams KF, et al. Short-term intravenous milrinone for acute exacerbation of chronic heart failure: a randomized controlled trial. JAMA. 2002;287:1541–7.
33. Felker GM, Benza RL, Chandler AB, et al. Heart failure etiology and response to milrinone in decompensated heart failure. J Am Coll Cardiol. 2003;41:997–1003.
34. Ramanathan K, Cosmi J, Harkness SM, et al. Reversal of systemic hypoperfusion following intra aortic balloon pumping is associated with improved 30-day survival independent of early revascularization in cardiogenic shock complicating an acute myocardial infarction. Circulation. 2003;108(suppl 1):I-672.
35. O'Gara PT, Kushner FG, Ascheim DD, et al. American College of Cardiology Foundation/American Heart Association Task Force on Practice Guidelines. 2013 ACCF/AHA guideline for the management of ST-elevation myocardial infarction: a report of the American College of Cardiology Foundation/American Heart Association Task Force on Practice Guidelines. Circulation. 2013;127(4):e362–426.
36. Chen EW, Canto JG, Parsons LS, et al. Investigators in the National Registry of Myocardial Infarction 2. Relation between hospital intra-aortic balloon counterpulsation volume and mortality in acute myocardial infarction complicated by cardiogenic shock. Circulation. 2003;108(8):951–7.
37. Urban PM, Freedman RJ, Ohman EM, et al. In-hospital mortality associated with the use of intra-aortic balloon counterpulsation. Am J Cardiol. 2004;94(2):181–5.
38. Hochman JS, Sleeper LA, Webb JG, et al. Early revascularization and long-term survival in cardiogenic shock complicating acute myocardial infarction. JAMA. 2006;295(21):2511–5.
39. Zeymer U, Vogt A, Zahn R, et al. Predictors of in-hospital mortality in 1333 patients with acute myocardial infarction complicated by cardiogenic shock treated with primary percutaneous coronary intervention (PCI); Results of the primary PCI registry of the Arbeitsgemeinschaft Leitende Kardiologische Krankenhausärzte (ALKK). Eur Heart J. 2004;25:322–8.
40. White HD, Assmann SF, Sanborn TA, et al. Comparison of percutaneous coronary intervention and coronary artery bypass grafting after acute myocardial infarction complicated by cardiogenic shock: results from the Should We Emergently Revascularize Occluded Coronaries for Cardiogenic Shock (SHOCK) trial. Circulation. 2005;112(13):1992–2001.
41. Sleeper LA, Ramanathan K. Picard MH, et al Functional status and quality of life after emergency revascularization for cardiogenic shock complicating acute myocardial infarction. J Am Coll Cardiol. 2005;46(2):266–73.
42. Kar B, Gregoric ID, Basra SS, et al. The percutaneous ventricular assist device in severe refractory cardiogenic shock. J Am Coll Cardiol. 2011;57(6):688–96.
43. Thiele H, Smalling RW, Schuler GC. Percutaneous left ventricular assist devices in acute myocardial infarction complicated by cardiogenic shock. Eur Heart J. 2007;28(17):2057–63.

4 Obstructive Shock

Kyung Su Kim

4.1 Introduction

4.1.1 Definition of Obstructive Shock

Obstructive shock is a form of shock associated with mechanical obstruction of blood flow to the heart, specifically left ventricle (Fig. 4.1) [1].

The most distinctive feature of obstructive shock is that detecting the cause of obstruction is essential for the proper management and the response to the treatment is very immediate. This section deals with following three conditions of obstructive shock: tension pneumothorax, pulmonary thromboembolism, and cardiac tamponade.

4.1.2 Common Pathophysiology of Obstructive Shock

The common pathophysiology of obstructive shock is a reduction in the left ventricular (LV) preload. Increased intrathoracic pressure impairs venous return in tension pneumothorax. Increased right ventricular (RV) afterload impairs blood flow from right to left heart in pulmonary embolism. Decreased cardiac compliance impairs diastolic filling of heart in cardiac tamponade. Decreased LV preload leads to the relative increase in both LV contractility and heart rate, but eventually the stroke volume and cardiac output (CO) decrease. Because of the obstruction of the blood flow, distended jugular vein and inferior vena cava (IVC) can be commonly observed in physical examinations or bedside sonography.

4.1.3 Initial Approach and Diagnosis of Obstructive Shock

Except for hypotension, the most common symptoms and signs of obstructive shock are dyspnea and jugular venous distension (Fig. 4.2). Also, venous congestion due to obstruction can be visualized by bedside sonography as distended hepatic inferior vena cava (IVC) without significant inspiratory collapse (Fig. 4.2).

Careful medical history and physical examination in unstable patients provide a valuable information to distinguish the cause of the shock. In addition, bedside ultrasonography is one of the most useful tools to identify causes of shock. The presence, location, and volume of pneumothorax can be diagnosed by the ultrasonography and RV strain on the ultrasonography can be a very important finding in suspicion of massive pulmonary embolism. In particular, the ultrasonography is the diagnostic tool of choice in pericardial tamponade and it can also guide the pericardiocentesis.

K. S. Kim
Department of Emergency Medicine, Seoul National University Hospital, Seoul, South Korea

G. J. Suh (ed.), *Essentials of Shock Management*, https://doi.org/10.1007/978-981-10-5406-8_4

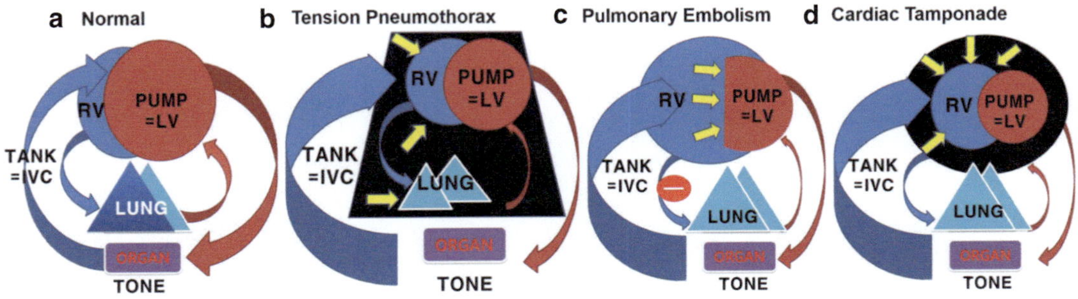

Fig. 4.1 Three types of obstructive shock. (**a**) Diagram describing the normal circulation. (**b**) Tension pneumothorax (Black) alters venous return, which results in decreased cardiac output and venous congestion. (**c**) Pulmonary embolism (Red prohibition sign) blocks the blood flow from right heart to left heart, which results in distension of right ventricle and diastolic septal flatening. (**d**) Cardiac tamponade (Black) compresses cardiac chambers, which results in decreased cardiac output and venous congestion. *RV* right ventricle, *LV* left ventricle, *IVC* inferior vena cava

Fig. 4.2 (**a**) Jugular venous distension and (**b**) distended hepatic inferior vena cava. *IVC* inferior vena cava, *HV* hepatic vein, *RA* right atrium

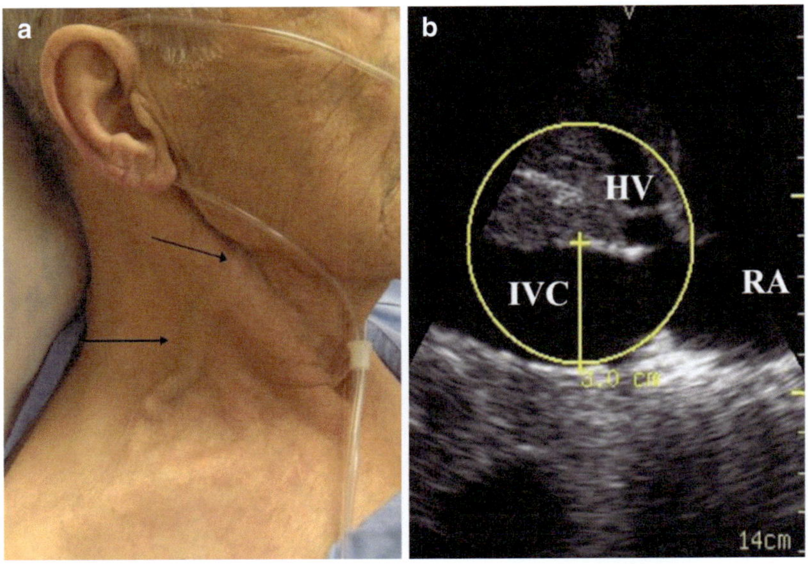

4.1.4 General Management of Obstructive Shock

Airway management is required in patients with decreased mentality or with profound shock. As described above, most patients with obstructive shock also suffer from hypoxemia. Therefore, supplement oxygen should be delivered in patients with hypoxemia. Ventilatory support may be required in respiratory-distressed patients. Volume resuscitation is the first step for the circulatory support. In patients with obstructive shock, venous system is similar to those with volume overload. Jugular vein and IVC are distended and central venous pressure and pulmonary artery occlusion pressure are elevated. However, their cardiac output still can respond to volume resuscitation because cardiac filling pressure is increased in obstructive shock. Of course, immediate identification and management of the obstructive lesion are essential for the outcome. If blood pressure is not recovered rapidly, vasopressors can be used empirically.

4.2 Tension Pneumothorax

4.2.1 Definition of Tension Pneumothorax

A tension pneumothorax is considered to be present when a pneumothorax leads to significant hemodynamic compromise [2].

4.2.2 Epidemiology of Tension Pneumothorax

The incidence of tension pneumothorax varies widely among the studies including trauma patients, performed in emergency departments, or in intensive care units [2]. Tension pneumothorax was diagnosed in 5.4% of major trauma patients in one study [3].

4.2.3 Pathophysiology of Tension Pneumothorax

Causes of tension pneumothorax include trauma, obstructive lung diseases (asthma, chronic obstructive pulmonary diseases), and excessive positive pressure ventilation. Once the lungs are injured leaked air is accumulated in the pleural cavity and cannot escape. Accumulated air increases intrathoracic pressure and finally obstructs venous return to the heart, which results in the obstructive shock. Ventilation-perfusion mismatch and decreased vital capacity due to collapsed lung contribute to hypoxemia and respiratory distress [2].

4.2.4 Initial Approach and Diagnosis of Tension Pneumothorax

Most patients with pneumothorax have acute pleuritic chest pain and increasing volume of pneumothorax causes dyspnea, hypoxemia, tachycardia, and hypotension. Common physical findings are tracheal deviation toward the contralateral side of tension pneumothorax, hyperresonance and diminished lung sounds on the affected side, subcutaneous emphysema, and neck vein engorgement. Persistent shock may result in the bradycardia and pulseless electrical activity arrest.

Diagnostic modalities for pneumothorax are chest radiography (Fig. 4.3), chest CT, and ultrasonography (Fig. 4.4). However, confirmative evaluation should not delay treatment for unstable patients suspected of tension pneumothorax.

4.2.5 Management of Tension Pneumothorax

The definite treatment of tension pneumothorax is the decompression of accumulated air in the pleural space. Immediate needle decompression is the treatment of choice in the emergent situation. A 14-gauge needle or larger should be placed over the superior margin of the third rib in the midclavicular line (Fig. 4.5). A rush of air with clinical improvement of vital signs confirms the diagnosis. If there is no immediate improvement, do not hesitate to place a second needle in the next interspace. The chest tube should be placed subsequently.

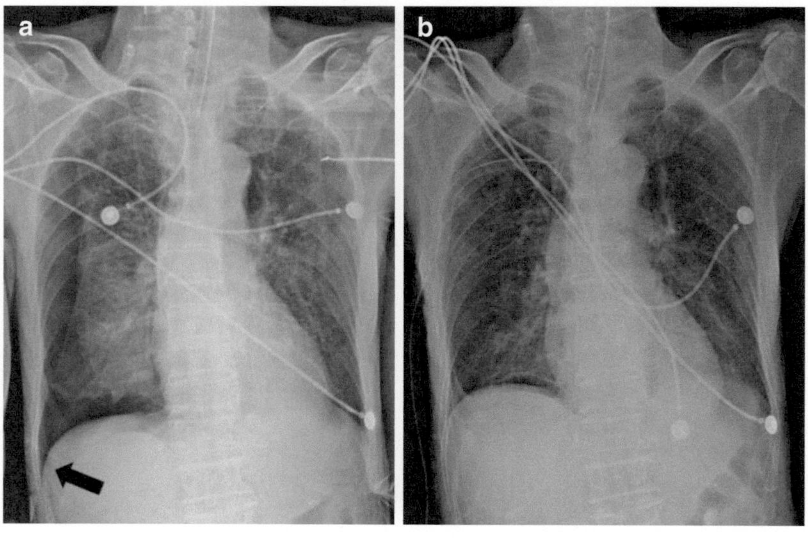

Fig. 4.3 (**a**) Pneumothorax in the right pleural cavity with deep sulcus sign (arrow). (**b**) Pneumothorax disappeared after tube thoracotomy

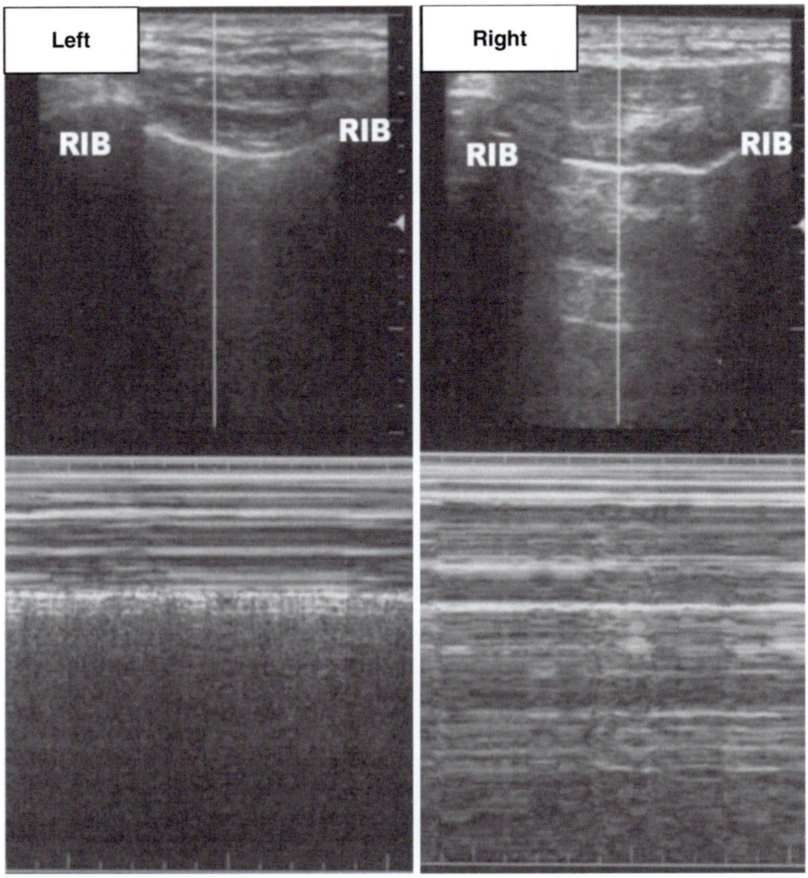

Fig. 4.4 M-mode image of bilateral lung. Left image shows normal seashore sign and right image shows stratosphere (bar code) sign indicating the presence of pneumothorax

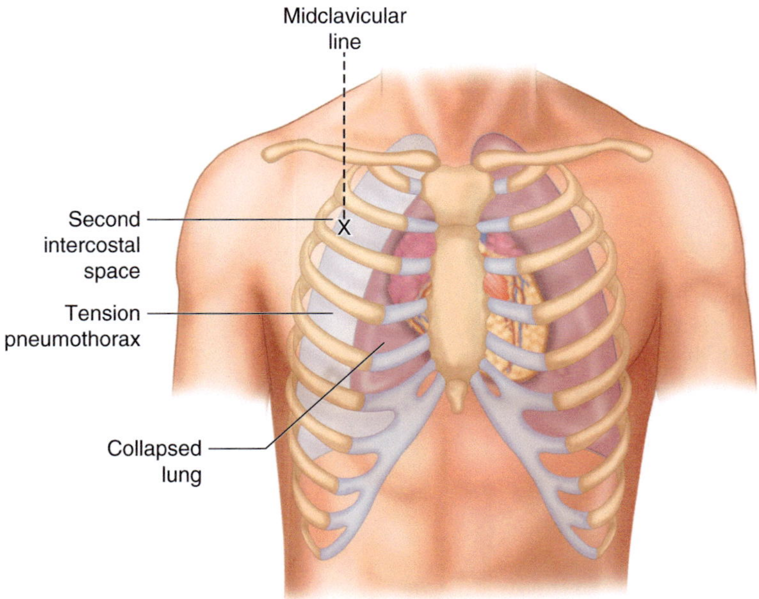

Fig. 4.5 Illustration of needle thoracotomy

4.3 Pulmonary Thromboembolism

4.3.1 Definition of Pulmonary Thromboembolism

Pulmonary thromboembolism is defined as a blockage of a pulmonary artery by the thrombus traveled mainly from veins of lower extremities [4]. Therefore, the term venous thromboembolism is used for both deep vein thrombosis and pulmonary thromboembolism.

4.3.2 Epidemiology of Pulmonary Thromboembolism

Venous thromboembolism occurs about ten million cases very year and this burden accounts for the third leading vascular disease following acute myocardial infarction and stroke [5].

4.3.3 Pathophysiology of Pulmonary Thromboembolism

Most common cause of pulmonary embolism is the thrombus from the deep veins of the lower extremities. Therefore, deep vein thrombosis and pulmonary thromboembolism compose of single disease entity, venous thromboembolism. Acute embolism of pulmonary artery leads to ventilation perfusion mismatch, which results in hypoxemia and dyspnea. If the thrombus obstructs a substantial portion of pulmonary artery, the increase in pulmonary vascular resistance impedes RV outflow and reduces LV preload and CO [4].

4.3.4 Initial Approach and Diagnosis of Pulmonary Thromboembolism

The symptoms and signs of pulmonary thromboembolism are usually nonspecific, making it difficult to diagnose. Therefore, pulmonary thromboembolism should be considered whenever unexplained symptoms including dyspnea, syncope, hypotension, and hypoxemia are present. D-dimer test has high negative predictive value to diagnose pulmonary thromboembolism and is widely used to exclude pulmonary thromboembolism. Because false-positive elevation of D-dimer is common in various conditions such as sepsis and malignancy, its positive predictive value is very low and further confirmatory diagnostic test is required. Wells' criteria are a clinical decision rule to provide the risk stratification for pulmonary embolism (Table 4.1) and pulmonary embolism rule-out criteria rule can be used (Table 4.2) [6, 7].

In patients with massive pulmonary thromboembolism and acute cor pulmonale, S1Q3T3 pattern can be observed in electrocardiography (ECG) (Fig. 4.6). However, this ECG changes are neither sensitive nor specific for pulmonary thromboembolism.

Table 4.1 Wells' score for pulmonary thromboembolism

Criteria	Points
Clinical signs and symptoms of deep vein thrombosis	3
Pulmonary embolism is most likely diagnosis	3
Tachycardia over 100 beats/min	1.5
Immobilization or surgery in previous 4 weeks	1.5
Prior diagnosis of deep vein thrombosis or pulmonary thromboembolism	1.5
Hemoptysis	1
Active malignancy	1

Low risk <2 points, intermediate risk 2–6 points, high risk >6 points
Pulmonary thromboembolism unlikely 0–4 points, likely >4 points

Table 4.2 Pulmonary embolism rule-out criteria rule (all nine factors must be present to exclude pulmonary embolism)

Clinical low probability (<15% probability of pulmonary embolism based on gestalt assessment)
Age <50 years
Pulse <100 beats/min during entire stay in ED
Pulse oximetry >94% at near sea level (>92% at altitudes near 5000 feet above sea level)
No hemoptysis
No prior venous thromboembolism history
No surgery or trauma requiring endotracheal or epidural anesthesia within the last 4 weeks

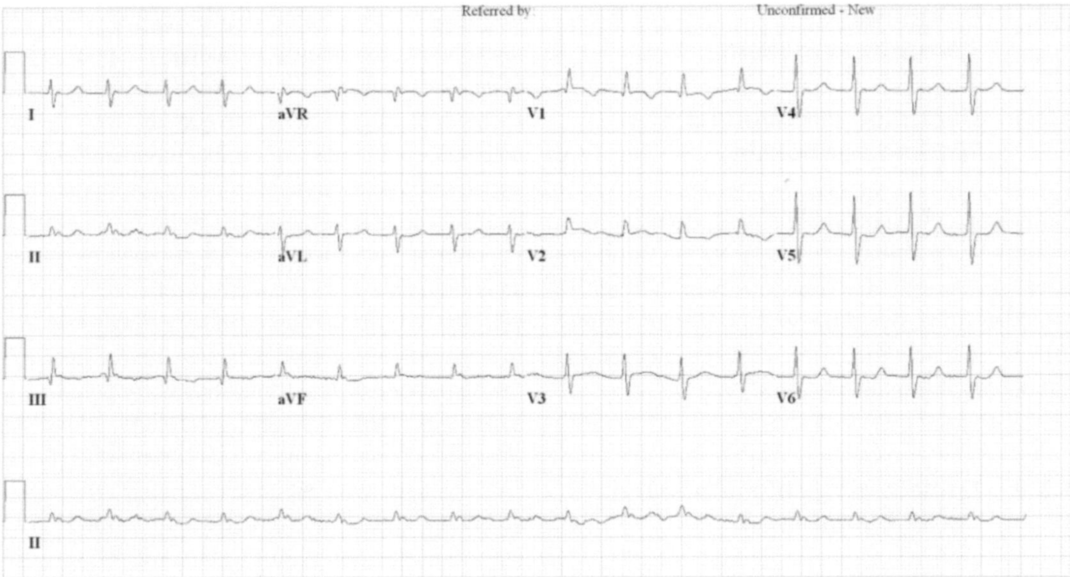

Fig. 4.6 Deep S wave in lead I, Q wave, and inverted T wave in lead III are classic findings of acute cor pulmonale

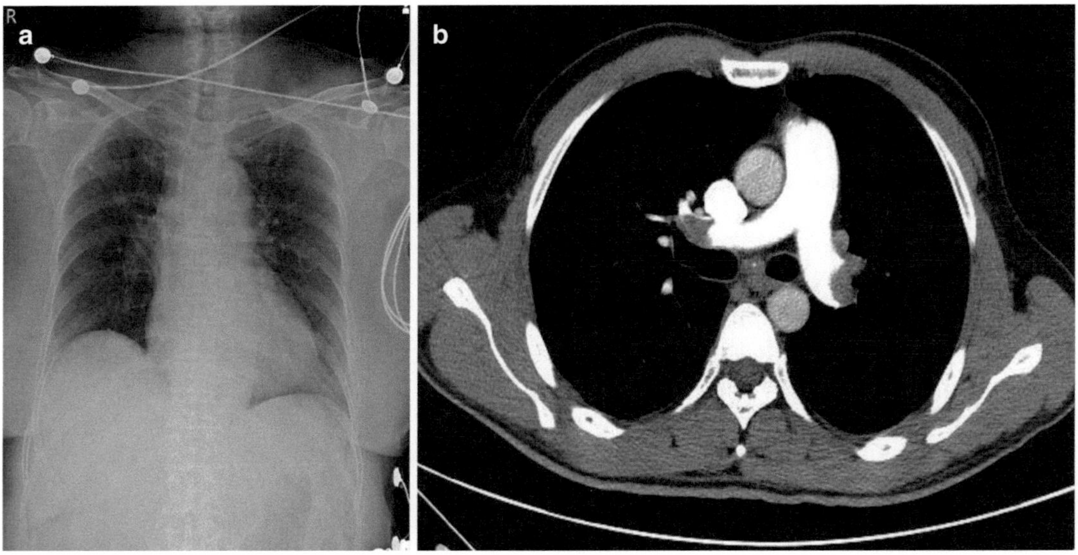

Fig. 4.7 (**a**) Chest radiography does not give any diagnostic information in pulmonary thromboembolism in most cases. (**b**) Bilateral main pulmonary arteries are occluded by thromboembolism in chest CT scan with contrast

In most cases, chest radiography does not give any diagnostic information in pulmonary thromboembolism (Fig. 4.7). For the confirmative diagnosis, chest CT scan with contrast or conventional angiography should be performed.

When pulmonary embolism is suspicious, the presence of deep vein thrombosis also should be excluded. Therefore, CT angiography protocol in many institutions includes the lower extremity venography by obtaining delayed phase of image.

Bedside ultrasonography can be helpful especially in patients with hemodynamic instability. Pulmonary thromboembolism can be directly visualized in pulmonary artery or right ventricle. Also, RV dilation and flattening of

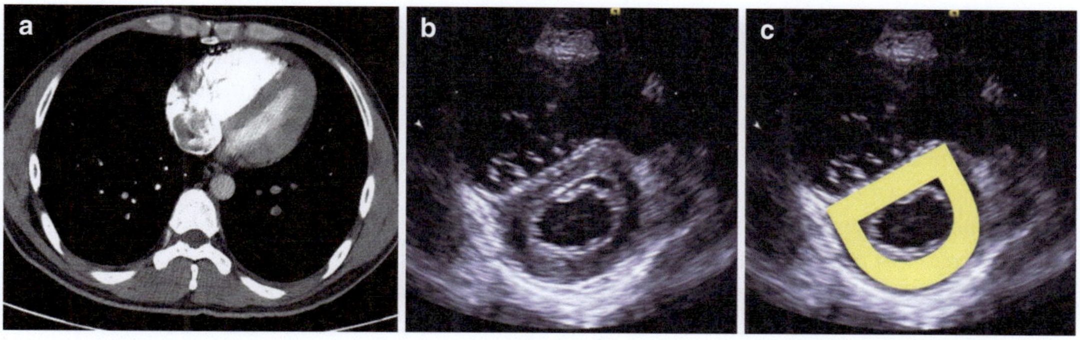

Fig. 4.8 (**a**) Chest CT shows RV dilation in massive pulmonary thromboembolism. Note that right ventricle is larger than left ventricle. (**b**, **c**) Typical D-shape left ventricle in massive pulmonary embolism is observed in parasternal short-axis view. Right ventricle is also larger than left ventricle indicating right ventricular dilation

interventricular septum (D-shape LV) can be seen especially in massive pulmonary thromboembolism with obstructive shock (Fig. 4.8). These findings are not sensitive enough to exclude pulmonary thromboembolism, but very specific to pulmonary thromboembolism if there is no history of chronic lung disease and pulmonary hypertension.

In addition, bedside ultrasound can detect proximal venous thrombosis using Doppler images and compression technique. Normal vein can be easily compressed by ultrasound probe. However, vein filled with thrombosis cannot be compressed by the probe.

Although CT angiography is more widely used nowadays, ventilation-perfusion lung scan can be helpful to diagnose the pulmonary embolism especially in patients with renal failure; in that circumstance the avoidance of radiocontrast dye is warranted.

4.3.5 Management of Pulmonary Thromboembolism

The primary treatment for pulmonary embolism is anticoagulant therapy, but since anticoagulant therapy does not lysate the thrombus immediately, thrombolytic therapy should be considered for severe cases of pulmonary embolism. The hemorrhagic complication rate of thrombolysis in pulmonary thromboembolism is higher than those in myocardial infarction and ischemic stroke because the burden of thrombosis is larger and consumptive coagulopathy is already present. Therefore, thrombolytic therapy is indicated in patients with high risk of death from pulmonary thromboembolism. In patients with life-threatening pulmonary embolism, thrombolysis should always be considered even in patients with relative contraindications. Meta-analysis which has evaluated the role of thrombolysis in pulmonary embolism showed that thrombolysis improves the all-cause mortality (1.39% vs. 2.92%, p value = 0.03) in intermediate-risk patients who were hemodynamically stable with RV dysfunction [8]. However, the rate of major bleeding events was significantly higher in thrombolysis group (7.74% vs. 2.25%, p value <0.001) in that study. One randomized clinical trial reported that thrombolysis could prevent hemodynamic decompensation but increased the risk of major hemorrhage and stroke in patients with intermediate-risk pulmonary embolism [9]. Because the hemorrhagic complication especially intracranial hemorrhage following thrombolysis therapy is usually catastrophic, the clinical benefit of thrombolysis in patients without hemodynamic instability is still controversial.

Two indications of thrombolysis in current guideline are acute massive pulmonary thromboembolism (high-risk pulmonary embolism, systolic blood pressure <90 mmHg, or a decrease in systolic arterial pressure of at least 40 mmHg for at least 15 min) and acute sub-massive pulmonary thromboembolism (intermediate-high risk, normal blood pressure with RV dysfunction) [10]. Thrombolysis regimen is the intravenous infusion of 100 mg of tissue-type plasminogen activator (tPA) during 2 h in the absence of contraindications. In cases who cannot tolerate anticoagulation therapy, inferior vena cava filter can be used to prevent further occlusion of pulmonary artery. Lastly, venoarterial extracorporeal membrane oxygenator (VA ECMO) can be considered in profound obstructive shock or cardiac arrest from pulmonary thromboembolism.

4.4 Cardiac Tamponade

4.4.1 Definition of Cardiac Tamponade

Cardiac tamponade is defined as an acute circulatory failure due to the compression of the cardiac chambers by the pericardial effusion.

4.4.2 Epidemiology of Cardiac Tamponade

The incidence of cardiac tamponade is not well documented because most epidemiological studies have examined patients suffering from a pericardial effusion without focusing on tamponade [11].

4.4.3 Pathophysiology of Cardiac Tamponade

Causes of cardiac tamponade include metastatic malignancy, pericarditis, uremia, and tuberculosis. As fluid accumulates within the pericardial sac, intrapericardial pressure increases. There are relatively small changes in the intrapericardial pressure in the early stage because of the distensibility of parietal pericardium. However, if the fluid continues to accumulate beyond the limits, the intrapericardial pressure increases rapidly. If the intrapericardial pressure rises over the normal RV filling pressure, ventricular filling is restricted and results in the decrease in the RV end-diastolic volume. The decreased RV end-diastolic volume compromises CO which results in obstructive shock.

4.4.4 Initial Approach and Diagnosis of Cardiac Tamponade

Early symptoms include dyspnea at rest and with exertion. Common physical findings are tachycardia, narrow pulse pressure (reflecting decreased stroke volume), and neck vein engorgement. Inspiratory decrease in systolic blood pressure may be observed and this is called pulsus paradoxus. The classic Beck triad includes jugular venous distension, hypotension, and muffled hear sounds.

Chest radiography may reveal an enlarged heart silhouette and epicardial fat-pad sign (Fig. 4.9).

ECG usually shows low-voltage QRS complexes and sometimes electrical alternans (beat-to-beat variation in the amplitude) (Fig. 4.10).

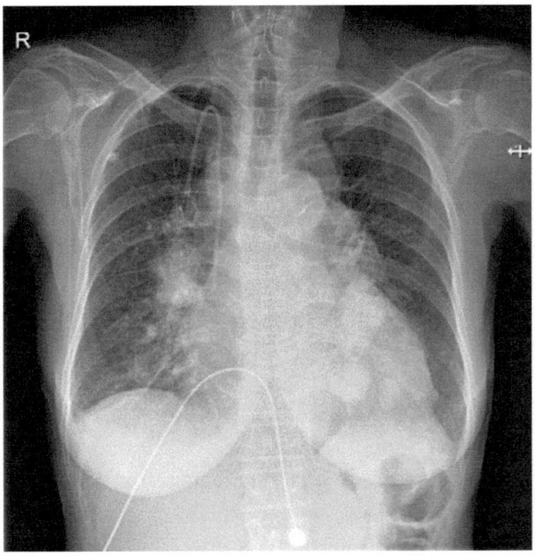

Fig. 4.9 Chest radiography of patient with malignant pericardial effusion

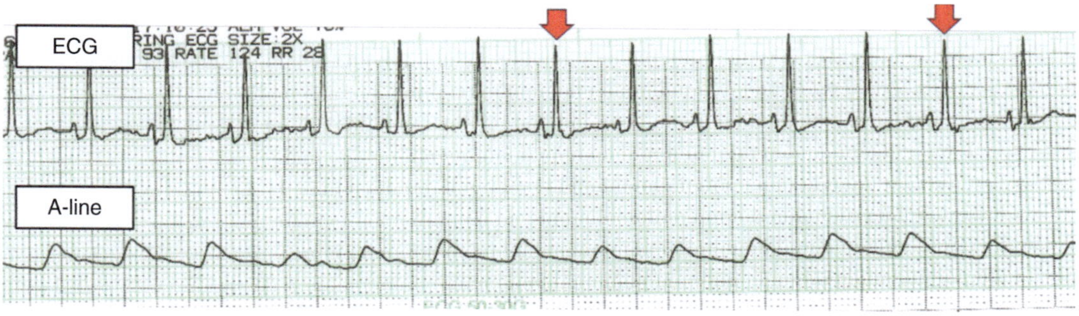

Fig. 4.10 Electrical alternans (beat-to-beat variation amplitude) is observed in patients with pericardial tamponade. Note that arterial wave also shows variation of size

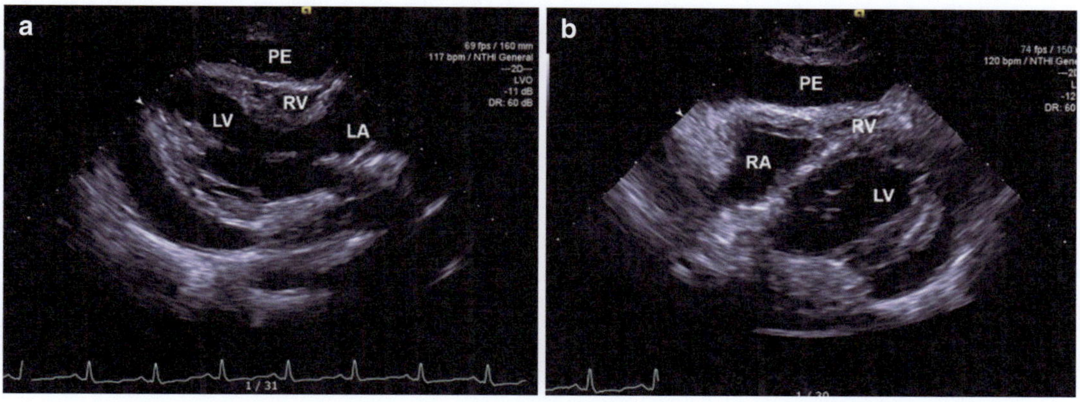

Fig. 4.11 Diastolic right ventricular collapse can be observed (**a**) in parasternal long-axis view and (**b**) in subxiphoid four-chamber view. *PE* pericardial effusion, *RV* right ventricle, *LV* left ventricle, *LA* left atrium

Echocardiography is the diagnostic test of choice. In addition to a large pericardial fluid volume, typical echocardiographic findings described in cardiac tamponade are right atrial compression, RV diastolic collapse, and dilated IVC with lack of inspiratory collapse (Fig. 4.11).

4.4.5 Management of Cardiac Tamponade

The primary treatment for cardiac tamponade is pericardiocentesis. If cardiac tamponade is suspected and the patient is not in cardiac arrest, expert consultation should take place. If cardiac arrest is ongoing or impending and cardiac tamponade is suspected, emergency pericardiocentesis should be performed. Pericardiocentesis is optimally performed using echocardiographic guidance to avoid cardiac perforation and coronary artery laceration (Fig. 4.12).

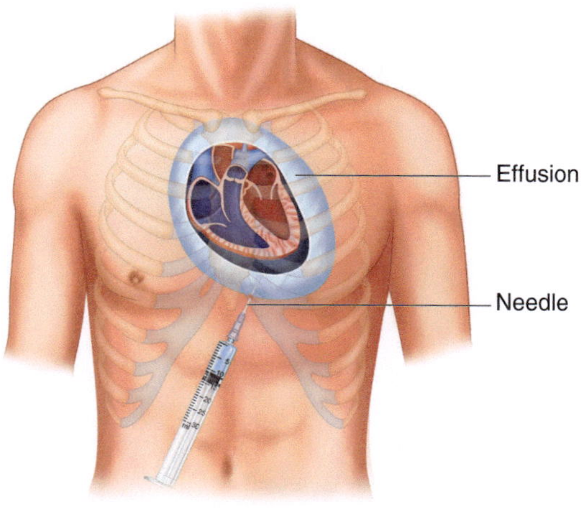

Fig. 4.12 Emergent pericardiocentesis for pericardial tamponade

References

1. McLean AS. Echocardiography in shock management. Crit Care. 2016;20:275.
2. Leigh-Smith S, Harris T. Tension pneumothorax—time for a re-think? Emerg Med J. 2005;22:8–16.
3. Coats TJ, Wilson AW, Xeropotamous N. Pre-hospital management of patients with severe thoracic injury. Injury. 1995;2:581–5.
4. Di Nisio M, van Es N, Büller HR. Deep vein thrombosis and pulmonary embolism. Lancet. 2016;388:3060–73.
5. Raskob GE, Angchaisuksiri P, Blanco AN, et al. Thrombosis: a major contributor to global disease burden. Arterioscler Thromb Vasc Biol. 2014;34:2363–71.
6. Wolf SJ, McCubbin TR, Feldhaus KM, Faragher JP, Adcock DM. Prospective validation of Wells Criteria in the evaluation of patients with suspected pulmonary embolism. Ann Emerg Med. 2004;44:503–10.
7. Kline JA, Courtney DM, Kabrhel C, et al. Prospective multicenter evaluation of the pulmonary embolism rule-out criteria. J Thromb Haemost. 2008;6:772.
8. Chatterjee S, Chakraborty A, Weinberg I, et al. Thrombolysis for pulmonary embolism and risk of all-cause mortality, major bleeding, and intracranial hemorrhage: a meta-analysis. JAMA. 2014;311:2414–21.
9. Konstantinides SV, Vicaut E, Danays T, et al. Impact of thrombolytic therapy on the long-term outcome of intermediate-risk pulmonary embolism. J Am Coll Cardiol. 2017;69:1536–44.
10. Konstantinides SV, Torbicki A, Agnelli G, et al. 2014 ESC guidelines on the diagnosis and management of acute pulmonary embolism. Eur Heart J. 2014;35:3033–69.
11. Bodson L, Bouferrache K, Vieillard-Baron A. Cardiac tamponade. Curr Opin Crit Care. 2011;17:416–24.

5 Septic Shock

Kyuseok Kim, Han Sung Choi, Sung Phil Chung, and Woon Young Kwon

5.1 Introduction

5.1.1 Definition

More than 20 years, sepsis was defined as symptoms associated with the response to microorganism infection, which was more specifically called systemic inflammatory response syndrome (SIRS). With the evidence of organ failure, it was called severe sepsis, and this could lead to hypotension (septic shock) [1]. However, with the deep understanding of the pathophysiology of sepsis, sepsis has been known as both inflammatory and anti-inflammatory. Additionally, the classic use of SIRS could lead to overestimation of sepsis. For example, usual common cold could be identified as sepsis in classic definition [2]. With this background, new sepsis definition, Sepsis 3, was introduced with expert consensus, literature review, and finally big data analysis. Sepsis was defined as a "life-threatening organ dysfunction caused by a dysregulated host response to infection." They recommended the use of sequential organ failure assessment (SOFA) score as clinical criteria for sepsis in ICU encounters. More specifically, increase in SOFA score of two points or more should be used. In non-ICU encounters, quick SOFA score was recommended as screening tool, and qSOFA score of two or more was set to identify high-risk patients. The concept of classical severe sepsis was eliminated. Septic shock was newly defined as sepsis with fluid-unresponsive hypotension, serum lactate level greater than 2 mmol/L, and need for vasopressors to maintain mean arterial pressure of 65 mmHg or greater (Fig. 5.1) [3, 4].

5.1.2 Epidemiology

Annual worldwide incidence of sepsis was estimated from 15–31 million, but this wide estimation stems from various methods used in calculation. This reflects vagueness and difficulty in sepsis definition. However, the incidence has

K. Kim (✉)
Department of Emergency Medicine, Seoul National University Bundang Hospital, Gyeonggi-do, South Korea

H. S. Choi
Department of Emergency Medicine, Kyung Hee University School of Medicine, Seoul, South Korea

S. P. Chung
Department of Emergency Medicine, Gangnam Severance Hospital, Yonsei University College of Medicine, Seoul, South Korea

W. Y. Kwon
Department of Emergency Medicine, Seoul National University College of Medicine, Seoul, South Korea

G. J. Suh (ed.), *Essentials of Shock Management*, https://doi.org/10.1007/978-981-10-5406-8_5

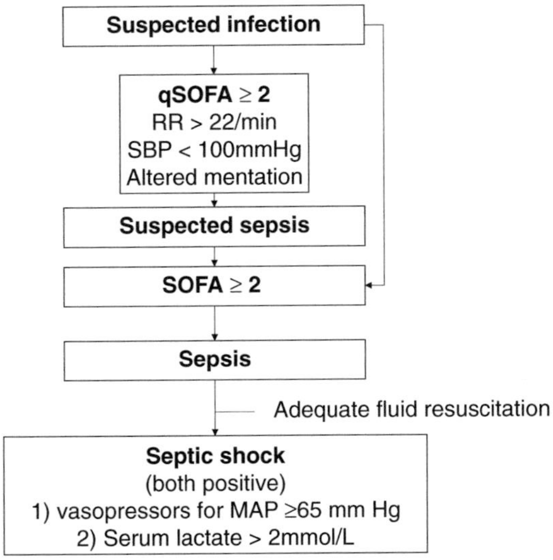

Fig. 5.1 Sepsis-3 Definition of sepsis and septic shock [4]

been investigated to increase as consistently, and aging and more comorbid disease (cancer, diabetes, etc.) may affect this increase [5, 6].

5.1.3 No Magic Bullet as a Drug in Septic Shock Treatment

High disease burden in respect to the incidence, morbidity, and mortality has led to the extensive research about the septic shock, but unfortunately no drug has survived from clinical trials. This could mean the poor understanding of pathophysiology, different subphenotypes, diverse phases, etc. [5]. With more knowledge of septic shock, it is rapidly changing how to manage the septic shock, which would be briefly discussed.

5.1.4 Introduction to This Chapter

In this chapter, we introduce the pathophysiology, diagnostic approach, initial management, and future of septic shock. Considering the purpose of this book, i.e., scenario based, we do not cover all aspects of septic shock, but focus on the early management of septic shock.

5.2 Pathophysiology of Septic Shock

5.2.1 Introduction

Although septic shock is one of the distributive shocks, the pathophysiology of septic shock is different from other distributive shock diseases. The pathophysiology and the clinical course of septic shock are more complex and vary over the course of the disease, with variable degrees of intravascular volume depletion, peripheral vasodilation, and cardiac dysfunction.

Septic shock can be produced by any microbial infection (bacteria, virus, fungus, parasites, etc.), even if no organism is identified at nearly 50% of cases of septic shock. Lipopolysaccharide (LPS) of gram-negative [G (−)] bacteria and lipoteichoic acid and peptidoglycan of gram-positive [G (+)] organisms are well-known mediators of sepsis.

5.2.2 Pathophysiology

5.2.2.1 Mediators

Against invading organism or its toxins, the early humoral responses are the complement system involvement and immune cell [monocytes/macrophages and polymorphonuclear neutrophils (PMNs), etc.] activation. Immune cells not only are able to recognize invading organisms and their products so they can destroy them but also release a series of mediators that can activate other cells. Toll-like receptors, among cell membrane receptors, are implicated in the recognition of pathogenic agents. Cellular stimulation activates intracellular signaling and results largely in the activation of transcriptional factors (including nuclear factor kappa B), which initiate proinflammatory reactions in turn. A number of cytokines, mainly tumor necrosis factor alpha (TNF-α) and interleukin (IL)-1, are released by macrophages and other cells. TNF-α and IL-1 are particularly important proinflammatory cytokines that can reproduce all features of septic shock including hypotension and development of multiple-organ

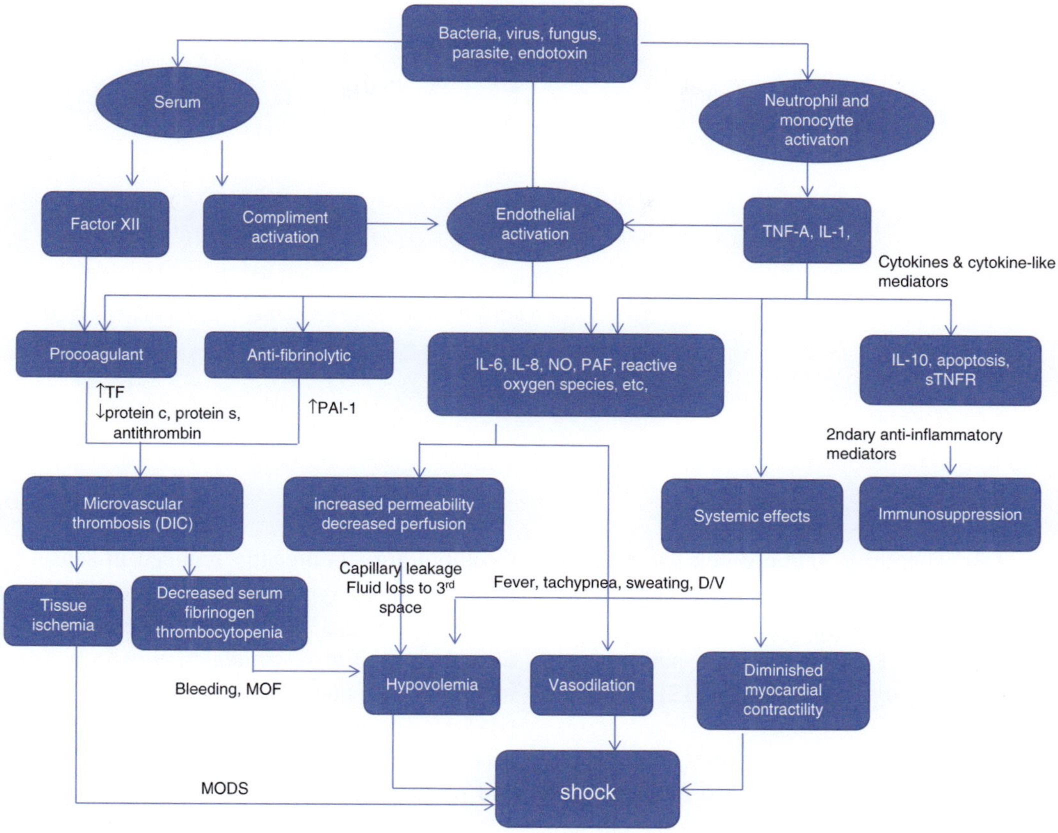

Fig. 5.2 The pathophysiology of septic shock

failure (MOF) in animal studies. Anti-inflammatory mediators including IL-4 and IL-10 are also released during the sepsis response, which limit the effects of proinflammatory mediators and can lead to a state of relative immunosuppression sometimes called immunoparalysis [7]. When sepsis is diagnosed, many patients are already immunosuppressed [8].

Immune cells also release secondary host mediators including lipid mediators, oxygen free radicals, proteases, and arachidonic acid metabolites. Vasodilator substances such as nitric oxide (NO) and prostaglandins are released by endothelial cells and are responsible for the early hemodynamic changes of sepsis. The formation of large quantities of NO can also have secondary toxic effects on cells. NO can block mitochondrial respiration, directly by inhibiting cytochrome a and a3 and reacting with superoxide radicals, resulting in the production of peroxynitrite, which inhibits various phases of mitochondrial respiration [9] (Fig. 5.2).

5.2.2.2 Hemodynamic Changes

Widespread systemic inflammation likely plays a role in the development and persistence of multisystem organ failure in sepsis through microvascular and mitochondrial dysfunction. Although microcirculatory and mitochondrial dysfunction in sepsis and its links with organ dysfunction are not fully understood, they are likely to be key locus of hemodynamic compromise in septic shock [10, 11]. Septic shock is often due to three major causes: intravascular volume depletion, cardiac dysfunction, and peripheral vasodilation. And they also may be associated with microcirculatory and mitochondrial dysfunction

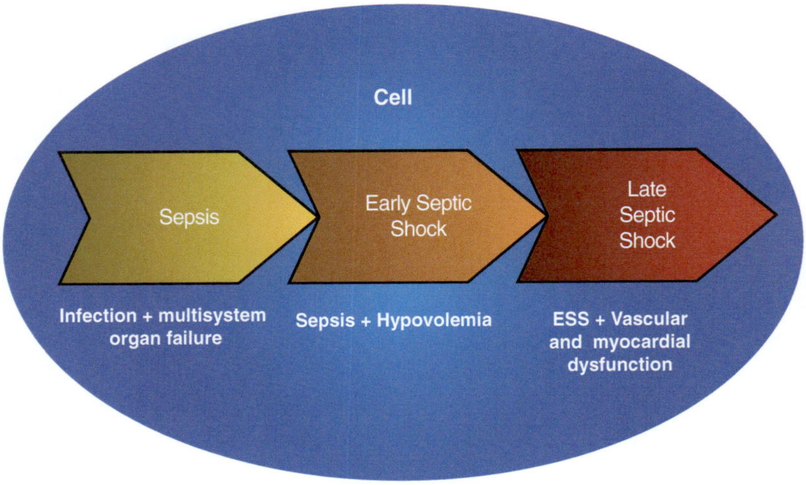

Fig. 5.3 The phase of septic shock

(Fig. 5.2). Therefore, septic shock was recently classified, according to pathophysiological background, into two stages as follows: the early hypovolemic and the late vascular and myocardial circulatory dysfunction stage [12] (Fig. 5.3).

Intravascular Volume Depletion

Sepsis produces hypovolemia, and the hypovolemia contributes partially to deterioration into septic shock. Hypovolemia in septic shock mainly results from gastrointestinal volume loss (diarrhea, vomiting), tachypnea, sweating, and decreased fluid intake during development of the illness.

The other auxiliary cause of hypovolemia in septic shock results from increasing capillary leak and resultant loss of intravascular volume into third spaces. In septic shock, adhesion molecules on vascular endothelium and circulating cells (platelets, PMNs, and monocytes) are expressed by inflammatory reaction. Activated leukocytes adhere to vascular endothelium and migrate to subendothelial tissues. Alterations in intercellular endothelial junctions result in increased capillary permeability and generalized edema [13].

Alterations in coagulation and fibrinolysis complete the picture, with proinflammatory mediators creating a procoagulant state. Briefly, the activation of tissue factor on the surface of various cells, particularly monocytes and endothelial cells, initiates the coagulation system [13]. Endotoxin, TNF-α, and IL-1 are the key mediators. The plasma levels of natural anticoagulants such as protein C, protein S, and antithrombin are significantly reduced in sepsis by reducing their synthesis and increasing their consumption and clearance. In early sepsis, thrombolysis is also stimulated with an increase in the levels of plasminogen activator inhibitor-1 (PAI-1). The net result is a balance in favor of procoagulant processes, often leading to DIC and participating in the microcirculatory disorder that leads to MOF in many patients with sepsis. This sequence of events leads to consumption of coagulation factors and the fibrinolytic system is suppressed in late sepsis and that promotes capillary leakage, bleeding, and third-space fluid shift (Fig. 5.2).

Cardiac Dysfunction

Cardiovascular dysfunction and failure arise from direct myocardial depression and distributive shock condition. Any microbes and killed organisms can cause myocardial depression. The direct effects of the toxic mediators as well as the knock-on effects of host mediators of sepsis produce a septic shock. Septic shock causes direct myocardial depression. Even in the hyperdynamic stages, cardiac contractility becomes impaired during the early phase of septic shock. Circulating mediators, inflammatory myocardial cellular injury, and deranged metabolism interact synergistically to injure the heart during septic shock, and specific cytokines (most notably TNF-α and IL-lß), overproduction of NO, and possibly impairment in mitochondrial respiration may contribute to the cardiovascular dysfunction.

Early in sepsis, although the cardiac output (CO) is increased, it is at the expense of ventricular dilation and decreased ejection fraction (EF). After vascular filling as a result of volume resuscitation, the hemodynamic status in septic shock is characterized by a fall in vascular tone associated with reduced systemic vascular resistance and a raised CO. Ejection volume and, particularly, CO may be maintained by an increase in diastolic volumes. Therefore, myocardial depression or dysfunction without any true cardiac failure would be developed and that may be associated with reduced cardiac output.

Peripheral Vasodilation

NO is a powerful vasodilator acting on vascular smooth muscle. Increased NO production in sepsis is essentially due to the induction of inducible NO synthase (iNOS) by proinflammatory cytokines. NO regulates vascular tone by an indirect effect on smooth muscle cells and that is important role in septic shock. NO also contributes to platelet adhesion, insulin secretion, neurotransmission, tissue injury, and cytotoxicity, and it seems to be a key mediator of septic shock although its mechanisms of action are not well understood. Enhanced NO production is thought to contribute to the profound vasodilation found in patients in septic shock.

Vasopressin is a naturally occurring hormone that is essential for cardiovascular stability. It is produced as a prohormone in the hypothalamus. The hormone is stored in the pituitary gland and released in response to stressors such as pain, hypoxia, hypovolemia, and hyperosmolality. There is a brief rise in circulating vasopressin levels in sepsis and followed by a prolonged and severe suppression in septic shock.

5.3 Septic Shock: Initial Approach and Diagnosis

5.3.1 Recognition of Sepsis Candidate

According to the new definition updated in 2016 published by "The Third International Consensus Definitions for Sepsis and Septic Shock" (Sepsis-3) in 2016, sepsis is a life-threatening organ dysfunction caused by a dysregulated host response to infection [4]. A clinical algorithm to identify patient with sepsis and septic shock was also proposed (Fig. 5.4). Sepsis screening is associated with earlier treatment because a lack of its recognition may prevent timely therapy [14]. A significant challenge in recognizing sepsis may be the complexity of the sepsis presentation. Notably, sepsis screening has been associated with survival improvement [15].

5.3.1.1 Patients with Suspected Infection

The above algorithm starts from patient with suspected infection, which may include a wide range of patients. A prospective cohort study showed that 13% of patients admitted to the intensive care unit (ICU) with suspected sepsis had in fact no infection identified [16]. Such sepsis mimickers are consisted of adverse drug reaction, acute mesenteric ischemia, malignancies, and various sterile inflammatory diseases [17]. The presence of an infectious process is by definition necessary to discriminate between sepsis and sepsis mimickers. However, patients with sepsis mimickers have a clinical phenotype that resembles that of patients with sepsis, so that antimicrobial agents are usually administrated within the first hours of recognition of shock, until infection is ruled out and an alternative noninfectious diagnosis is made.

5.3.1.2 Quick SOFA Score

The quick Sepsis-related Organ Function Assessment (qSOFA) score was introduced as an initial screening tool to screen sepsis, which comprises a respiratory rate of 22/min or greater, altered mentation, or systolic blood pressure of 100 mmHg or less. If a patient has at least two of these criteria present, he or she could be identified as being more likely to have poor outcome of sepsis [4]. A patient with a qSOFA score of 2 or higher had a 3- to 14-fold increase in hospital mortality compared with a patient with a qSOFA score lower than 2 [18]. Compared with previous SIRS criteria, qSOFA had better discriminative value and hazard ratio for predicting death, ICU admission, and ICU stay longer than 72 h.

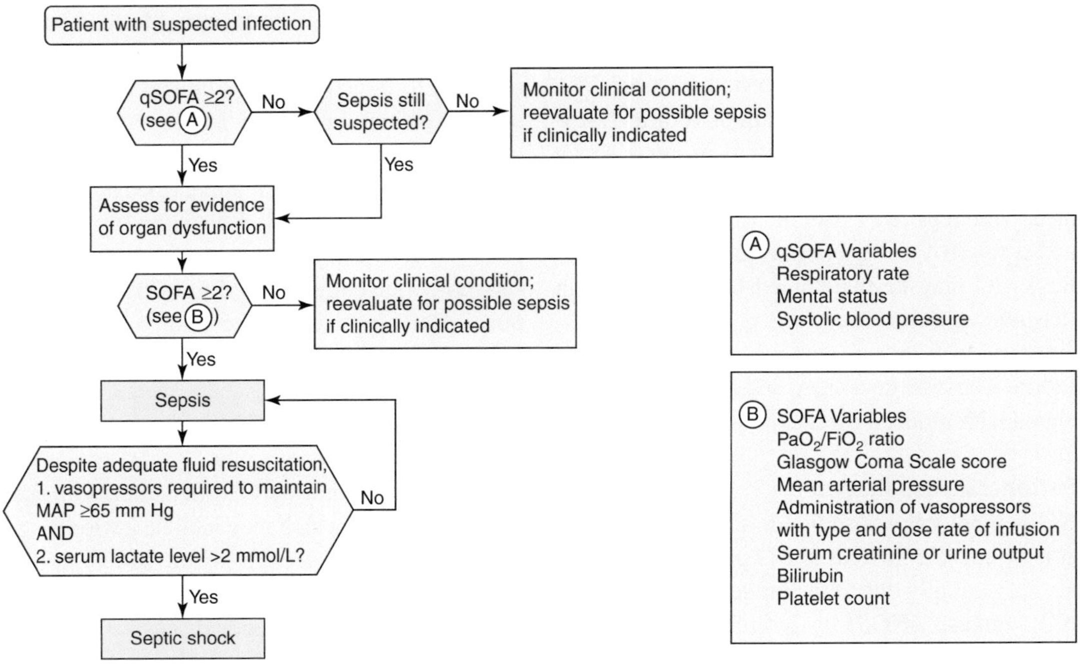

Fig. 5.4 Operationalization of clinical criteria identifying patients with sepsis and septic shock. SOFA: Sepsis-related Organ Function Assessment. Modified from ref. [4]

The strong prognostic accuracy of qSOFA for mortality was confirmed with an area under the receiver operating characteristic (AUROC) of 0.80, which was greater than that of SIRS and severe sepsis (AUROC 0.65 for both) [19]. However, a recent prospective study reported that a qSOFA score of two or higher had high specificity for organ dysfunction but poor sensitivity (96.1% vs. 29.9%, respectively) [20].

5.3.1.3 Other Screening Tools

Many other potential clinical scoring systems could be used as a screening tool including simple triage scoring system (STSS), rapid emergency medicine score (REMS), modified early warning score (MEWS), and national early warning score (NEWS). They are easy to use because they only require simple physiological measures such as heart rate, blood pressure, respiratory rate, oxygen saturation, mental status, and urine output. These variables can easily be measured in primary care setting.

Several studies based on electronic screening tools have been reported in order to recognize sepsis without delay. A prospective observational study showed that an electronic alert was sent to the care team if two or more SIRS criteria were detected in patients older than 70 years. The system had a sensitivity of 14% and a specificity of 98% for detecting an infection [21]. Nelson et al. used an automated messaging system that alerted the care team if a patient presented to the ED with two or more SIRS criteria in addition to two systolic blood pressure readings of <90 mmHg. Their system had a sensitivity of 64% and specificity of 99% [22]. Sepsis performance improvement programs can be aimed at earlier recognition of sepsis via a formal screening effort and improved management of patients once they are identified as being septic.

5.3.2 Organ Dysfunction Assessment

The Sepsis-3 algorithm recommends to assess for evidence of organ dysfunction using the SOFA score for a patient with suspected sepsis who has a qSOFA score of two or higher. The SOFA score is based on six different scores, consisted of the respiratory, cardiovascular, hepatic, coagulation, renal, and neurological systems. A SOFA score of two points or more is associated with an in-hospital mortality greater than 10% and is therefore considered indicative for a patient with suspected infection having sepsis.

Besides SOFA score, there are some potential scores to assess organ dysfunctions in the emergency department setting such as Mortality in Emergency Department, Sepsis (MEDS); Confusion, Urea nitrogen, Respiratory rate, Blood pressure, 65 years and older (CURB-65); predisposition, infection, response, and organ dysfunction (PIRO); Acute Physiology and Chronic Health Evaluation (APACHE) scores; and Simplified Acute Physiology Score (SAPS) are more complicated scores to calculate, as they require for example the measurement of arterial oxygenation; therefore they are usually used in critical care settings. These scores could be used as a prognostic indicator to estimate the mortality of critically ill patients.

5.3.3 Clinical Manifestations

The septic patient may manifest signs of systemic infection. The symptoms and signs of sepsis are nonspecific but may include the following: temperature >38.3 or <36 °C, heart rate >90 beats/min, respiratory rate >20 breaths/min, and arterial hypotension (systolic blood pressure <90 mmHg or mean arterial pressure <70 mmHg). Symptoms and signs may be various and specific to an infectious source. For example, cough or dyspnea may suggest pneumonia, and pain and purulent exudate in a surgical wound may suggest an underlying abscess.

Warm, flushed skin may be present in the early phases of sepsis. As sepsis progresses to shock, the skin may become cool due to redirection of blood flow to core organs. Decreased capillary refill, cyanosis, or mottling may indicate shock. Additional signs of hypoperfusion include altered mental status, obtundation or restlessness, and oliguria or anuria. Ileus or absent bowel sounds are often an end-stage sign of hypoperfusion. These findings may be modified by preexisting disease or medications. For example, older patients, diabetic patients, and patients who take beta-blockers may not exhibit an appropriate tachycardia as blood pressure falls. In contrast, younger patients frequently develop a severe and prolonged tachycardia and fail to become hypotensive until acute decompensation later occurs. Patients with chronic hypertension may develop critical hypoperfusion at a higher blood pressure than healthy patients (relative hypotension). Importantly, the presentation is nonspecific such that many other conditions such as pancreatitis and acute respiratory distress syndrome may present similarly.

5.3.4 Adequate Fluid Resuscitation

By definition of Sepsis-3, the identification of patients with septic shock includes the requirement of vasopressors to maintain a mean arterial pressure of 65 mmHg or greater and the presence of serum lactate levels greater than 2 mmol/L despite adequate fluid resuscitation [4]. Therefore, we need to administrate adequate fluid to identify the patients with septic shock as well as shock management.

5.3.4.1 Controversy for EGDT

Early effective fluid resuscitation is crucial for stabilization of sepsis-induced tissue hypoperfusion or septic shock. Sepsis-induced hypoperfusion may be manifested by acute organ dysfunction and/or decreased blood pressure and increased serum lactate. Previous guidelines have recommended a protocolized quantitative resuscitation, also known as early goal-directed therapy (EGDT) [23]. This approach has been challenged following the failure to show a mortality reduction in large RCTs such as ARISE, PROCESS, and PROMISE trial [24–26]. Although, the EGDT protocol cannot now be recommended from its evidence base, bedside clinicians still need guidance as to how to approach patients suspicious of septic shock who have significant mortality and morbidity.

5.3.4.2 Volume of Fluid for Initial Resuscitation

Surviving Sepsis Campaign (SSC) guideline recommended that these patients be viewed as having a medical emergency that necessitates urgent assessment and management [27]. As part of this, guideline recommends that initial fluid resuscitation begin with 30 mL/kg of crystalloid within the first 3 h. This fixed volume of fluid enables clinicians to initiate resuscitation while obtaining more specific information about the patient and while awaiting more precise measurements of hemodynamic status. The average volume of fluid before randomization given in the PROCESS and ARISE trials was approximately 30 mL/kg, and approximately 2 L in the PROMISE trial [24–26].

5.3.4.3 Optimal Fluid Type for Initial Resuscitation

The optimal fluid in the initial resuscitation of sepsis is not yet clear. Solutions containing water and freely permeable ions, mainly sodium and chloride, are classified as crystalloids. Balanced solutions are usually defined as intravenous fluids having an electrolyte composition close to that of plasma. Balanced crystalloids such as Plasma-Lyte solution are probably superior to normal saline, but further prospective studies are warranted [28].

Albumin appears to be equivalent to crystalloids in terms of outcomes, but should be second-line due to higher cost. Among patients with sepsis, several randomized trials and meta-analyses have reported no difference in mortality when albumin was compared with crystalloids, although one meta-analysis suggested benefit in those with septic shock [29–31]. In the Saline versus Albumin Fluid Evaluation (SAFE) trial performed in critically ill patients, there was no benefit to albumin compared with saline even in the subgroup with severe sepsis, who comprised 18% of the total group [32]. Hydroxyethyl starches (HES) appear to increase mortality and acute kidney injury in critically ill septic patients and are no longer indicated in the treatment of this patient population. In the Scandinavian Starch for Severe Sepsis and Septic Shock (6S) trial, compared with Ringer's acetate, use of HES resulted in increased mortality (51% vs. 43%) and renal replacement therapy (22% vs. 16%) [33]. There is very limited clinical data regarding the use of hypertonic saline and no data regarding the use of plasma in sepsis.

5.3.5 Assessment of Fluid Responsiveness

Unnecessary fluid administration in the treatment of shock can increase morbidity and mortality, whereas selective yet timely use of fluids has shown to be beneficial. For adequate fluid resuscitation, physicians should assess the fluid responsiveness which is the ability of cardiac output to increase in response to a fluid infusion. Static measures of preload such as filling pressures and volumes are poor predictors of fluid responsiveness. The use of CVP alone to guide fluid resuscitation can no longer be justified because the ability to predict a response to a fluid challenge when the CVP is within a relatively normal range (8–12 mmHg) is limited [34].

Therefore, dynamic indices which measure the hemodynamic response of the cardiovascular system to a controlled variation in preload have been introduced in clinical practice. The most investigated dynamic indices such as the pulse pressure variation measure the response to preload variations induced by mechanical ventilation. They are good predictors of fluid responsiveness, but they lose their value in patients with spontaneous breathing activity and arrhythmias.

5.3.5.1 Passive Leg-Raising Test

To overcome the above limitations, the passive leg raising (PLR) has been proposed as an alternative preload-modifying maneuver. PLR induces a rapid, reversible increase in biventricular preload through an increase in venous return mimicking fluid administration. The reported amount of volume "autotransfused" by PLR ranges from 250 to 350 mL. Although PLR induces an increase in cardiac preload with its maximum effect at approximately 1 min, the effect is not sustained and vanishes completely when the legs are returned to the horizontal position. Thus, the hemodynamic effects of PLR must be assessed during a time frame of 30–90 s with a fast-responding method. No difference in diagnostic performance of PLR was seen in spontaneously breathing patients compared with controlled mechanically ventilated patients. Therefore, PLR has been proposed as an attractive way to predict fluid responsiveness and showed good diagnostic accuracy in meta-analysis [35]. The pooled sensitivity and specificity of PLR-induced changes in cardiac output were 89.4% (84.1–93.4%) and 91.4% (85.9–95.2%), respectively.

5.3.6 Serum Lactate Measurement

According to the Sepsis-3 definition, presence of serum lactate levels greater than 2 mmol/L is a component to diagnose septic shock. The 3-h bundle protocol recommends measurement of the serum lactate level to complete within 3 h. Serum lactic acid levels have long been identified as a diagnostic tool for global tissue hypoxia and therefore can serve in identifying patients with sepsis. However, increases in the serum lactate level may represent accelerated aerobic glycolysis driven by excess beta-adrenergic stimulation, or other causes including liver failure. Regardless of the source, increased lactate levels are associated with worse outcomes [36]. Several randomized controlled trials have evaluated lactate-guided resuscitation of patients with septic shock [27, 37, 38]. A significant reduction in mortality was seen in lactate-guided resuscitation compared to resuscitation without lactate monitoring (RR 0.67; 95% CI, 0.53–0.84). There was no evidence for difference in ICU length of stay (mean difference −1.51 days; 95% CI, −3.65 to 0.62).

5.3.6.1 Lactate Clearance

Another meta-analysis demonstrated reduction in mortality when an early lactate clearance strategy was used, compared with either usual care or a $ScvO_2$ normalization strategy [39, 40]. The lactate clearance was defined by the equation $[(lactate_{initial} - lactate_{delayed})/lactate_{initial}] \times 100\%$, for which $lactate_{initial}$ was the measurement at the start of the resuscitation and $lactate_{delayed}$ was another measurement after a minimum of 2 h after resuscitation was initiated [38]. It was shown that lactate clearance greater than 10% from initial measurement during the first 2–6 h of resuscitation predicted survival from septic shock and that protocols targeting lactate clearance of at least 10% produced similar short-term survival rates to protocols using $ScvO_2$ monitoring [38, 41]. Moreover, it was demonstrated that for every 10% increase in lactate clearance, there was a corresponding 11% decrease in in-hospital mortality [42]. Similarly, septic patients with lactate clearance of greater than 20% during the initial 8 h of resuscitation had a 22% decline in the relative risk of mortality, compared with patients having lactate clearances of less than 20% [37]. However, there was no association between degree of lactate clearance and change in microcirculatory blood flow in patients with septic shock [43].

5.3.7 Laboratory Findings of Sepsis

An ideal biomarker can be objectively measured and could play a role in sepsis screening, early diagnosis, risk stratification, critical assessment, and prognosis prediction. Numerous biomarkers have been studied for use in diagnosis or prognosis for sepsis. They consist of cytokines, cell markers, receptors, coagulation markers, acute-phase proteins, markers related to vascular endothelial damage, vasodilation and organ dysfunction, and so on [44]. Until now more than 170 different biomarkers have been assessed for potential use in sepsis. Several studies have proposed that measurement of multiple cytokines such as TNF-α, IL-1β, and IL-6 correlates well with disease severity and prognosis of sepsis. However, most of the cytokines and inflammatory mediators were of limited use in clinical setting.

5.3.7.1 C-Reactive Protein

The C-reactive protein (CRP) was identified as a protein responsible for precipitating C polysaccharide during the acute phase of *Streptococcus pneumonia* infection. Its response is stronger in acutely ill patients; levels decrease as patients recover. These characteristics make CRP a member of the class of acute-phase reactants. CRP is an old biomarker and widely used in clinical settings. It is a nonspecific marker of inflammation that also increases after surgery, burns, myocardial infarctions, and rheumatic diseases. According to a meta-analysis, the sensitivity and specificity of CRP as a marker for bacterial infections are 81% and 67%, respectively [45]. Its low specificity and inability to differentiate bacterial infections from noninfectious causes of inflammation make CRP of limited diagnostic value. However, CRP shows promise for evaluating sepsis severity and prognosis. CRP plasma levels have been shown to correlate with the severity of infection [46]. A rapid decrease in CRP levels has been reported to correlate with good response to initial antimicrobial therapy in septic patients [47]. CRP is a useful biomarker to monitor treatment response. However, CRP is not recommended to use in the day of sepsis diagnosis as a marker of prognosis and risk stratification [48].

5.3.7.2 Procalcitonin

Procalcitonin (PCT) is a precursor of calcitonin, a calcium-regulatory hormone secreted from thyroid tissue in healthy individuals. In infectious conditions, PCT is released from all tissues including lung, liver, kidney, pancreas, and adipose tissues. In a systematic review, PCT was found to be more specific (specificity 81%) than CRP (67%) for differentiating bacterial infection among hospitalized patients [45]. The cutoff value of PCT for diagnosis of sepsis has not yet been fully determined. PCT values need to be further evaluated according to different sites of infection, hosts, and pathogens. Another recent meta-analysis showed that PCT is a useful marker for early diagnosis of sepsis in critically ill patients, with sensitivity and specificity of 77% (95% CI: 72–81%) and 79% (95% CI: 74–84%), respectively [49]. PCT levels are also elevated after surgery, cardiogenic shock, heat shock, acute graft-versus-host disease, and immunotherapy such as granulocyte transfusion, which could limit its usefulness as a sepsis biomarker.

5.3.7.3 Antibiotic Stewardship with Procalcitonin

PCT has also drawn attention because it can be used for guidance of antibiotic stewardship to reduce inappropriate use of antibiotics [50]. Procalcitonin-guided therapy is defined as initiation of antibiotic treatment using PCT measurements, usually using a suggested treatment algorithm based on the height of the PCT measurement. Many studies used a cutoff of 0.25 ng/mL to suggest or encourage the initiation of antibiotics [51]. Multiple studies have investigated whether a PCT-guided algorithm can optimize the therapeutic approach in sepsis patients, mainly by monitoring PCT kinetics and stopping antibiotics once PCT has dropped to levels <0.5 ng/mL or by at least 80–90% of the peak in combination with clinical improvement. A meta-analysis including 1075 patients with sepsis or septic shock found overall reduced antibiotic treatment courses (6 days vs. 8 days) when PCT was used to guide therapy compared to routine care. There was no increase in 28-day or in-hospital mortality or in length of stay in the ICU or the hospital. The authors do stress that there was heterogeneity in PCT protocols across trials with regard to different cutoff values or different algorithms for medical or surgical patients [52]. A large RCT evaluated the use of PCT to de-escalate and stop antibiotics in critically ill patients who had received antibiotics <24 h before inclusion in the study for an assumed or a proven infection. The study found that the PCT-guided protocol shortened length of antibiotic treatment (5 days vs. 7 days in the first 28 days of admission) and lowered 28-day mortality from 25% to 19.6% [53].

5.3.8 Microbiologic Cultures

Blood cultures should be obtained prior to initiating antimicrobial therapy if cultures can be obtained in a timely manner. Several retrospective studies have suggested that obtaining cultures prior to antimicrobial therapy is associated with improved outcome [54]. However, the identification of an organism in culture in a patient with suspected sepsis is highly supportive of the diagnosis but is not necessary. The rationale behind its lack of inclusion in the diagnostic criteria for sepsis is that a culprit organism is frequently not identified in up to 50% of patients who present with sepsis nor is a positive culture required to make a decision regarding treatment with empiric antibiotics. Therefore, the desire to obtain cultures prior to initiating antimicrobial therapy should be balanced against the mortality risk of delaying a definitive therapy in patients with suspected sepsis or septic shock who are at significant risk of death [55].

Appropriate microbiologic cultures should be obtained before initiation of antimicrobial therapy from all sites considered to be potential sources of infection if it results in no substantial delay in the start of antimicrobials. This may include blood, cerebrospinal fluid, urine, wounds, respiratory secretions, and other body fluids. Two or more sets (aerobic and anaerobic) of blood cultures are recommended before initiation of any new antimicrobial in all patients with suspected sepsis [56]. All necessary blood cultures may be drawn together on the same occasion. Blood culture yield has not been shown to be improved with sequential draws or timing to temperature spikes [57].

5.4 Management of Septic Shock

5.4.1 Initial Resuscitation

1. Basal concept
   - To optimize tissue perfusion within 6 h post-diagnosis
   - To acquire the balance between the oxygen consumption (VO_2) and the oxygen delivery (DO_2) within 6 h post-diagnosis, but there have been no methods to estimate VO_2 during the acute phase of sepsis [27]. Therefore, the acute management of sepsis should be focused to increase DO_2 [58]. The formula to calculate DO_2 is as follows:

     $$DO_2 \approx CO \times 1.34 \times [Hb] \times SaO_2$$
   - To increase DO_2, cardiac output, hemoglobin concentration, and arterial oxygen saturation should be increased [59]. When adequate oxygen is provided, an increase in cardiac output can be a primary target for an increase in DO_2.
   - Cardiac output is calculated by stroke volume multiplied by heart rate. And the three components which contribute to make a stroke volume are preload, afterload, and myocardial contractility. Therefore, the basal concept of initial management to acquire optimal cardiac output is to maintain optimal preload, afterload, and contractility with an appropriate range of heart rate within 6 h post-diagnosis [23].

1.1. First Preload Optimization
   - The definition of preload for shock management is the end-diastolic volume of left ventricle. Preload is affected by venous pressure and venous return [60].
   - To increase venous return, first of all, adequate hydration (30 mL/kg of crystalloid) should be provided within 3 h [27].
   - To estimate volume status, many parameters are monitored. Because the direct measurement of left ventricular volume is impossible, most of the parameters monitor pressure. Commonly used parameters are static pressures which reflect left ventricle end-diastolic pressure. If the pulmonary circulation system would be intact, central venous pressure (CVP) is well correlated with pulmonary capillary wedge pressure (PCWP) and left ventricular end-diastolic pressure [61]. Because of the ease of accessibility and safety, CVP is the most commonly used parameter for static volume status in clinical setting [62]. However, many of the critically ill patients have structural or functional problems in pulmonary circulation system; CVP plays a limited

role in the estimation of acute-phase volume status in patients with septic shock [63, 64]. And thus, alternative parameters including the diameter and/or collapsibility of inferior vena cava (IVC) are tested [65, 66].
  - Initial hydration is the most important process to optimize preload and acquire appropriate tissue perfusion. But overhydration which induces fluid overload resulting in tissue edema and additional microcirculatory dysfunction should be avoided [67, 68]. Previous studies reported that fluid overload contributed to an increase in the mortality of patients with septic shock [69]. Therefore, the repeated measurements of dynamic fluid responsiveness should be combined with the measurement of static volume status.
  - The parameters monitoring static volume status have another limitation. They cannot reflect dynamic fluid responsiveness during initial resuscitation [61]. Therefore, adjunctive methods to predict dynamic fluid responsiveness, such as pulse pressure variation (PPV > 13%), stroke volume variation (SVV > 12%), passive leg raising (PLR), and mini-fluid challenge (stroke volume index >6% after 100 mL of fluid challenge), have been developed and applied [70–76]. Among them, PPV and SVV should be measured in patients with full sedation and positive pressure ventilation and without dysrhythmia, and the use of them in emergency department is limited [71–74].
  - The estimation of volume status and fluid responsiveness during fluid resuscitation is not easy in clinical setting. The combination of various monitoring parameters using all of the presently available devices may be helpful to estimate volume status more accurately and to optimize preload in patients with septic shock.

1.2. Second After Optimization
  - The definition of afterload for shock management is the pressure in the wall of the left ventricle during ejection. If aortic valvular function is maintained a systemic vascular resistance contributes to afterload to maintain blood flow to peripheral tissues.
  - To maintain systemic vascular resistance, the infusion of vasopressors is recommended.
  - Vasopressor should be infused after the optimization of preload. Previous studies showed that when vasopressors were infused before optimal hydration, the risk of patients' mortality increased [77–79].
  - To estimate afterload, mean arterial pressure (MAP) is commonly used. To measure more reliable MAP values, a routine intra-arterial catheterization in radial artery is recommended in patients with septic shock [27].

1.3. Third consider myocardial contractility augmentation with an appropriate range of heart rate
  - Myocardial contractility is the innate ability of the myocardium and an energy-consuming process. Furthermore, tachycardia also aggravates the energy-consuming process in myocardium. These energy-consuming processes need high oxygen supply to maintain the balance between VO_2 and DO_2.
  - In the current guideline, the routine use of inotropic agents is not recommended. Recent large clinical studies have shown that the routine use of inotropic agents does not contribute to the survival improvement of septic shock patients [24, 25, 80].
  - However, in patients who have acquired optimal preload and afterload but still have low cardiac output, the use of inotropic agents may be considered under the monitoring of stepwise changes in tissue perfusion with inotropic agents and heart rate [27].

1.4. Hemoglobin
  - To transport oxygen to peripheral tissues, adequate hemoglobin level should be maintained. There have been controversies about the optimal target hemoglobin level. When hemoglobin concentration is

15.0 g/dL, only a half of circulating hemoglobin participates in oxygen transport [81]. Furthermore, recent large clinical studies have shown that a transfusion threshold of the hemoglobin level of 7.0 g/dL was not different from 9.0 g/dL in the mortality of patients with septic shock [25, 82].

– Therefore, the current guideline recommends an erythrocyte transfusion threshold of 7.0 g/dL in patients with septic shock in the absence of myocardial infarction, severe hypoxemia, or acute hemorrhage [27, 83].

5.4.2 Surviving Sepsis Campaign Bundle

To optimize tissue perfusion with 6 h post-diagnosis, the current guideline recommends bundle therapies which should be completed within 3 h and 6 h, respectively (Table 5.1) [27, 84].

Table 5.1 Surviving sepsis campaign bundle

To be completed within 3 h	Measure lactate level
	Obtain blood culture prior to administration of antibiotics
	Administer broad-spectrum antibiotics
	Administer 30 mL/kg crystalloid for hypotension or lactate ≥4 mmol/L
To be completed within 6 h	Apply vasopressors for hypotension that does not respond to initial fluid resuscitation to maintain MAP ≥65 mmHg
	Remeasure lactate if initial lactate was elevated
	In persistent arterial hypotension despite volume resuscitation or initial lactate ≥4 mmol/L, RE-access volume status and tissue perfusion and document findings according to
	Repeat focused exam with respect to vital signs including mental status, cardiopulmonary including urination, capillary refill, pulse including tachycardia, and skin findings such as mottled skin
	Or two of the following: (1) Measure CVP: at least ≥8 mmHg (2) Measure ScvO2: ≥70% (3) Bedside cardiovascular ultrasound (4) Dynamic fluid responsiveness with PLR or mini-fluid challenge

5.4.3 Fluid Therapy

– Until now, the current guideline recommends the use of crystalloid for initial fluid resuscitation in patients with septic shock rather than colloid. Many previous studies reported that the use of colloid during initial resuscitation induces acute kidney injury and increases the mortality in patients with septic shock [33, 85].

– The current guideline recommends the use of crystalloid, both the 0.9% saline and the balanced crystalloids, such as Ringer's lactate solution and Plasma-Lyte. However, some studies showed that because of hyperchloremic metabolic acidosis, balanced crystalloids may be better than 0.9% saline for initial resuscitation (Table 5.2) [86, 87].

Table 5.2 Common crystalloids

	Plasma	0.9% saline	Ringer's lactate	Plasma-Lyte
Sodium (mmol/L)	136–145	154	130	140
Potassium (mmol/L)	3.5–5.0	0	4	5
Magnesium (mmol/L)	0.8–1.0	0	0	1.5
Calcium (mmol/L)	2.2–2.6	0	3	0
Chloride (mmol/L)	98–106	154	109	98
Lactate (mmol/L)	0	0	28	0

– To optimize preload, adequate fluid therapy should be provided. However, a sustained positive fluid balance after initial resuscitation has been reported to be harmful [88, 89]. Therefore, after preload optimization, fluid therapy should be cautiously performed with various monitoring devices to estimate the present volume status of patients.

– Although there have been no data supporting the amount of fluid volume after the 30 mL/kg of initial fluid resuscitation in patients with septic shock, the 30 mL/kg of initial fluid resuscitation, check volume status, additional fluid challenge (500 mL q 30 min) till CVP reaches ≥8 mmHg, recheck volume status with 100 mL of mini-fluid challenge, 150 mL of fluid infusion, and repeating the 100 mL of mini-fluid challenge and 150 mL of fluid infusion may be helpful to acquire optimal volume status.

- Recent clinical studies have shown the benefits of 5% albumin administration [32, 90]. Albumin administration can reduce fluid balance in septic shock patients who require substantial amounts of crystalloids. However, in patients with severe pneumonia or brain pathologies, the routine use of albumin should be avoided because the leakage of albumin can induce edema in lung or brain resulting in clinical deterioration [32].

5.4.4 Vasoactive Agents

- After optimized preload, to maintain afterload (MAP ≥65 mmHg) and cardiac contractility, vasoactive agents can be added. The commonly used vasoactive agents and their properties are described in Table 5.3 [91].
- The current guideline recommends to use norepinephrine as the first-choice vasopressor [27]. In previous studies, dopamine might induce tachyarrhythmia and deteriorated clinical outcomes in critically ill patients [92–94]. Therefore, dopamine can be considered for highly selected patients with low risk of tachyarrhythmia and absolute or relative bradycardia.
- If with the maximal dose of norepinephrine MAP failed to reach >65 mmHg, low doses of vasopressin or epinephrine can be added to norepinephrine [95, 96]. Vasopressin acts not to α-receptor but to V-receptor, and the deficiency of vasopressin may contribute to the vasodilation of septic shock [97]. The use of vasopressin can be helpful to decrease norepinephrine dosage.
- The use of dobutamine may be considered only in patients with persistent hypoperfusion despite adequate administrations of fluids and vasopressors [24, 25, 80].

5.4.5 Antimicrobial Therapy

- Antibiotics are the most important factor to improve survival in patients with septic shock. Particularly, IV antibiotics should be administered within 1 h after presenting symptoms and signs of septic shock [98, 99].
- We suggest the following three principles for the use of antibiotics in the emergency department for patients with septic shock.
  (1) Blood culture samples should be acquired before antibiotics administration. And thus, blood culture should be done within 45 min after presenting symptoms and signs of septic shock so as NOT TO delay antibiotics administration [27].
  (2) Accelerating appropriate antimicrobial therapy may cause a delay in the start of antibiotic therapy [100]. The combination therapy of two or more of broad-spectrum antibiotics should be provided as an empiric antimicrobial therapy. Then, according to the identified pathogens and clinical improvement, the empiric antimicrobial therapy should be de-escalated.
  (3) Imaging studies should be considered to find infection source, and if indicated invasive source control including radiologic interventions and/or surgery should be performed as soon as possible (within 12 h presenting symptoms and signs of septic shock).

Table 5.3 Common vasoactive agents

	Heart	Vasculature					Dose range
Agents	β1	α1	α2	Cardiac output	MAP	HR	(μg/kg/min)
Dopamine	0–3+	0–3+	0–2+	↑	↑	↑↑	2–20
Dobutamine	4+	1+	2+	↑↑	↔	↑	2.5–10.0
Epinephrine	4+	2–4+	1–3+	↑↑	↑↑	↑↑	0.005–0.200
Norepinephrine	2+	4+	1+	↔	↑↑	↑	0.04–1.00
Vasopressin	Vasopressin receptor			↓	↑	↔	0.01–0.04 U/min

5.4.6 Others

1. Glucose control:
   – To avoid hypoglycemic events, the target upper blood glucose level should be maintained ≤180 mg/dL [101].
2. Corticosteroid:
   – In recent large clinical studies, a routine use of corticosteroid failed to improve survival in patients with septic shock [102, 103]. Corticosteroid showed a benefit in the reversal of shock in patients who did not achieve hemodynamic stability in spite of adequate fluid resuscitation and vasopressor therapy [103].
   – The current guideline recommends IV hydrocortisone at a dosage of 200 mg/day with a continuous infusion rather than intermittent infusion to avoid a glucose fluctuation induced by corticosteroid administration [104, 105].

5.4.7 Summary

See Fig. 5.5

5.5 Future of Sepsis Management

5.5.1 Introduction: Current Problem of Sepsis Management

5.5.1.1 Definition/Epidemiology

The challenge for the management of sepsis might be originated from the "vagueness" of definition of sepsis. For a long time, the sepsis has been considered as one identity, which proved to be wrong. The sepsis could not be a "disease," but a simple symptom or response to more specific diseases, e.g., pneumonia, urinary tract infection, and biliary infection. Antibiotics treatment for sepsis should be

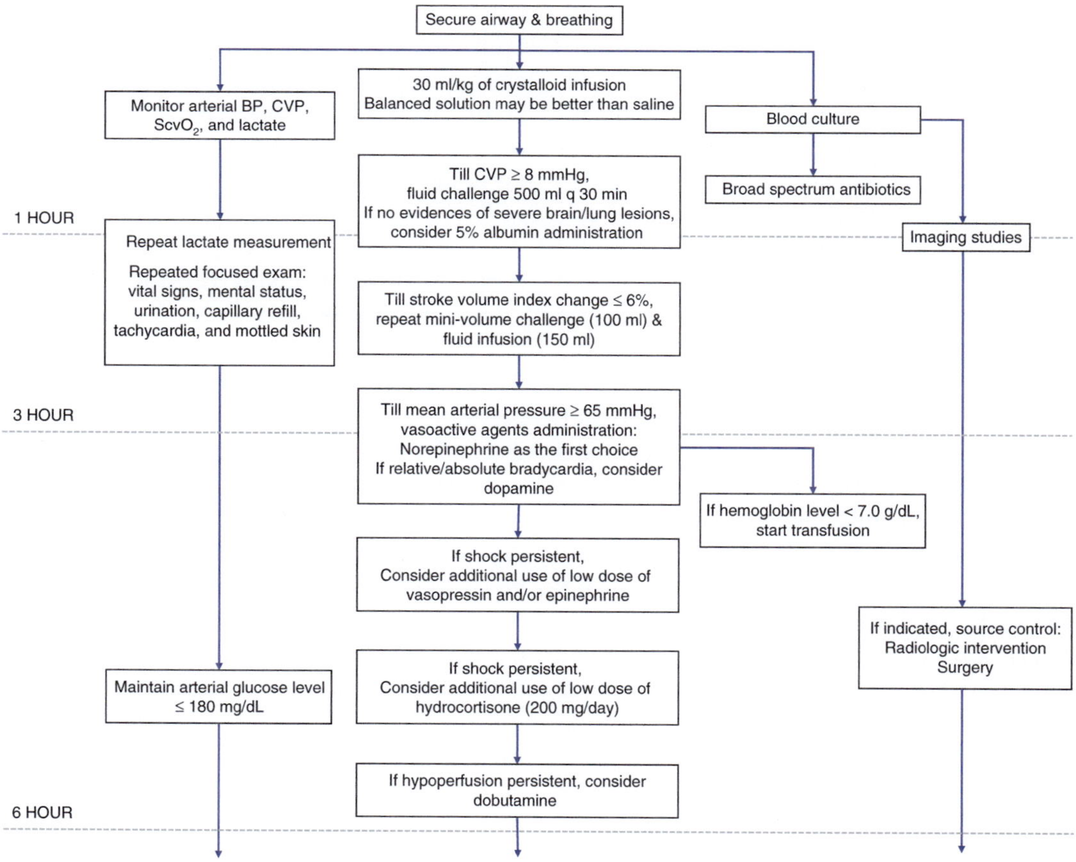

Fig. 5.5 Initial management of septic shock

different according to the severity, site of infection, or organisms of resistance. Other treatments of sepsis, such as vasopressor, steroid, and immune-targeting drugs, should also be chosen to specific conditions of sepsis. Taken together, sepsis should not be managed with one magic bullet even though some basic management (for example, early fluid management) could be same.

The wide epidemiologic range of sepsis over the world or even in same country could also be explained by various definitions of sepsis, which could make it difficult to see the trend or effect of treatment when tested in large clinical trials.

5.5.1.2 Preclinical Study: In Vitro/In Vivo Study

No drug has survived in final clinical trials, although many preclinical studies showed promising results. The gap could be explained in many aspects. The species-specific pathway of sepsis could be one reason. Usually, mouse has been used to see the effects of drugs or pathway of sepsis, and although many pathways are same in both rodents and humans there are different pathways or their significances between rodents and humans, which could make little translation into clinical outcome [106]. Also, the design of preclinical study should be mentioned. For example, lipopolysaccharide (LPS) model has little chance to be translated into human study [107]. No patients visit to the emergency department with LPS injection. With this background, recently the cecal ligation and puncture model has gained popularity. However, the diverse method used in this model could affect the translation, and efforts to standardize the method are under progress (Minimum Quality Threshold in Pre-clinical Sepsis Studies, MQTiPSS). Considering cecal ligation and puncture model, the animals usually get the fluid and antibiotics [107]. In real clinical situation, however, we perform source control and administer vasopressor, or ventilator care, if necessary as well as just one-shot antibiotics and fluid [108]. These affect clinical course dramatically. In these days, a few research centers run mouse or rat ICU, and this might help translation of preclinical research to clinical practice.

5.5.1.3 Phase and Severity

As mentioned above, the phase and severity of sepsis are definitely different among sepsis patients. One drug could be beneficial in phase A, but not or even harmful in phase B. One good example could be steroid [109]. If patients are in hyperinflammatory status, it could work, but in opposite situation it could be harmful. The use of vasopressin in septic shock is also interesting. As shown in VAAST trial, vasopressin could be beneficial in less severe septic shock without effects in more severe one [95].

5.5.1.4 Clinical Trial Design

Recently, previous clinical trial design has been challenged. Clinical trial design should reflect the real world, not just digging the statistics or so. With this background, more realistic design is emerging, i.e., platform trial or REMAP trial [110]. ACCESS trial has already adopted this design, and we hope this shows paradigm shift in the design of clinical trial.

5.5.2 Protocol-Based Bundle Management

5.5.2.1 Early Recognition: EMS/ED

Previously, and maybe nowadays, the management of sepsis has been ICU based. Now we understand that the early management of sepsis is mandatory. Supranormal oxygen delivery concept by Dr. Shoemaker failed [111], but the nearly same concept, early goal-directed therapy (EGDT) by Dr. Rivers, has saved many septic patients all over the world [23]. Actually, EGDT is the early application of supranormal oxygen delivery. We should manage the patients not in irreversible condition, which could already occur in ICU. Likewise, the management of sepsis could start in EMS or even at home. To do that, we should implement the early recognition and management protocol, which could be used in prehospital setting, or at home.

5.5.2.2 Fluid Management

Appropriate Fluid

Fluid resuscitation in sepsis is the mainstay in sepsis management. However, the issues regarding which fluid is more appropriate should be determined. Usually balanced crystalloids are favored [86, 87, 112, 113], but the pitfall of these fluids should be overcome, e.g., potassium containment. The role of albumin should be more specified since the current guideline is a little confusing (albumin could be used after "substantial" amount of crystalloid, but what is the definition of "substantial"?) [27]. However, this could be hard to prove in current clinical design [114], and again we need another platform of clinical study.

How Much Amount of Fluid?

Classically, preload has been measured with central venous pressure or pulmonary capillary wedge pressure, which has proved to be inappropriate parameters. Current recommendation for determining preload status (passive leg raising, dynamic parameters, such as pulse pressure variation, stroke volume variation, ultrasonographic parameters, or small volume challenges) has pros and cons [115], and the optimal and feasible method to see the fluid responsiveness should be explored with the more advanced technology.

5.5.2.3 Target Goal of Hemodynamics

Recently, the important clinical study showed that the target blood pressure in sepsis is between mean arterial pressure of 65 and 85 mmHg [116]. However, shown in this study, in chronic hypertension patients, the 80–85 mmHg target could be more optimal. Simple and unique target of blood pressure in sepsis has little chance of reflecting the optimal tissue perfusion, and in that sense individualized approach is ideal, which is not available in current practice. To achieve this, new technologies to monitor the optimal tissue perfusion directly should be investigated and validated.

5.5.3 Antibiotics

5.5.3.1 Initial Appropriate Antibiotics: Organism Isolation

Early appropriate administration of antibiotics is of paramount importance in sepsis management [27, 117]. The choice of appropriate antibiotics needs the identification of the specific microorganism. Currently, the isolation of organism takes a long time. With classical blood or body fluid culture, it takes at least 2–3 days [118], which could determine the fate of septic patients. More disappointingly, the yield of blood culture is not high [119]. Recently, the genome-based detection method has been introduced, but the diagnostic performance was not yet satisfied. A new method to isolate the specific microorganism or even resistant species is being investigated, but currently not in clinical use.

5.5.3.2 Maintenance Duration

The use of antibiotics has disadvantages such as rising resistant organisms and antibiotics-associated secondary infection. Determining the optimal duration of antibiotics is of great concern in this aspect. Currently, predetermined duration of antibiotics administration or the use of clinical information, e.g., fever, or some biomarker (CPR, procalcitonin), has been advocated [120–122], but not in a sufficient way. New biomarker-based approach is of need to be developed.

5.5.3.3 New Antibiotics

Recently, and rapidly, the multidrug-resistant bacteria have emerged over the world. The new super-antibiotics for these nagging bacteria are desperately necessary. Also, various, life-threatening viral infections need to have attention, but there are little antiviral agents.

5.5.4 Biomarker or Phenotype-Driven Management: Personalized Management

Sepsis is one of the perfect targets for the precision medicine. Sepsis is a group of diverse infected patients, and has dynamic change during short time. This means it needs a different approach from other diseases, such as cancer. In cancer, single measurement of subphenotype could lead to the specific treatment, but, in sepsis, the status could be different between today and tomorrow, or even change within hours. Considering that, the immediately available biomarker for specific conditions is of paramount importance. Even though not in sepsis, the opposite response to treatment according to the subphenotype of ARDS is very intriguing and could show the insight into sepsis management [123]. The effect of high PEEP or conservative fluid management was opposite with different subphenotypes in ARDS study, and this was validated using another big network sample [124]. Interestingly, the different subphenotypes were determined with inflammatory/anti-inflammatory cytokines, which have been used to see the phase of sepsis for a long time. Taken together, the same approach should be implemented in sepsis, and this approach could have huge impact on future sepsis management.

5.5.5 Promising Novel Therapeutic Strategies

5.5.5.1 New Vasopressor

Vasopressin

In VAAST trial, the use of vasopressin compared to norepinephrine showed no difference in survival. However, in less shock patients, the use of vasopressin showed lower mortality [95]. In substudy, the combined use of steroid proved to be more beneficial. Vasopressin in sepsis should be more investigated in two aspects. One is in less severe septic shock, and another is to use vasopressin as hormone, not just as vasopressor. Vasopressin showed bimodal secretion in many stressful situations, such as shock [125]. Vasopressin has many functions depending on the type of receptors. Sepsis is a stressful condition, and the role of vasopressin as stress hormone could have more effects than only as vasopressor. Regarding this, the strategy to use the continuous constant use of vasopressin as hormone and optimizing norepinephrine as vasopressor could be beneficial in sepsis.

Selepressin

Selepressin is the new selective V1a receptor agonist, and this drug has been investigated in septic shock, showing promising results. Currently phase 2b/3 clinical trial has been in progress [126].

Angiotensin II

Recent randomized clinical trial has been successfully performed to see the effects of angiotensin II in refractory to high-dose vasopressor. The primary outcome (MAP response) was achieved, and without statistical significance the trend to better survival was shown [127]. A larger trial would be anticipated.

5.5.5.2 Endothelial Homeostasis

Endothelial homeostasis has been known to be important in sepsis. Global increased permeability syndrome represents endothelial breakage and this could lead to multiple-organ dysfunction [128], which is the main concern of sepsis. The drug to maintain the endothelial homeostasis could lead to less organ injury, and finally survival benefit. For example, recently developed angiopoietin II antagonist showed dramatic effects on sepsis outcomes in preclinical study [129].

5.5.5.3 Immune Suppressor/Enhancer

Historically, the drugs to suppress cytokine storm have been used to treat sepsis. However, all drugs failed [130, 131]. This might not mean that there is no role in immune suppressor, but specific time point to use immune suppressor is mandatory. With biomarkers, we could define the status of septic patients whether the patients are under hyper-inflammation or immune paralysis. With this information, we could use immune suppressor or enhancer as appropriate. Recent study showed beneficial effect of immunostimulants [132] and many trials to use these agents are under investigation.

5.5.5.4 Mitochondrial Target

Mitochondria have gained much attention in sepsis. Mitochondria are very important in both bioenergetics and ROS production. Mitochondrial dysfunction or cytopathic hypoxia is one of the most important pathophysiologies of late sepsis [133]. Mitochondria-targeted treatment needs monitoring of mitochondrial function, and this could be real time based since the cellular status of sepsis changes dynamically, or superdynamically. There is no clinically available device for this purpose, but it is under investigation. The target of drug to maintain the function of mitochondria could be in control of mPTP opening, mitochondrial ROS scavenger, specific respiratory complex chain, etc.

5.5.5.5 Sympathetic/Parasympathetic Intervention

Brain and immune system has been known to be closely connected, especially via cholinergic pathway. Autonomic interventions to treat sepsis have been intensively investigated [134], but no drug or intervention has clinical translation. However, in the near future, it could be used. For example, esmolol in sepsis had promising clinical results [135], and we could see the results of large clinical trial.

5.5.5.6 Stem Cell

Likewise in other areas of medicine, stem cell research has been extensively under way in sepsis. For example, mesenchymal stromal cell has been studied and showed some beneficial effects [136], and the various mechanisms were proposed (direct effects, paracrine effects, extracellular vesicles, etc.). More extensive research is expected to investigate the effects of stem cells on the outcomes in sepsis.

5.5.6 Sepsis: From Vital Sign to Brain

Sepsis-associated long-term cognitive dysfunction has been investigated and the results are a little shocking [137]. Mild Alzheimer disease-level dysfunction has been shown, and the effects are diverse from medical to socioeconomic aspect. To target the brain resuscitation in sepsis, the extensive pathophysiologic studies should be done, and this area is underdeveloped. Recently, the hippocampus could be an important area in sepsis-associated cognitive impairment, and less dendrite in CA1 was implicated as an important pathophysiology [138].

References

1. American College of Chest Physicians. Society of Critical Care Medicine Consensus Conference: definitions for sepsis and organ failure and guidelines for the use of innovative therapies in sepsis. Crit Care Med. 1992;20(6):864–74.
2. Jacob JA. New sepsis diagnostic guidelines shift focus to organ dysfunction. JAMA. 2016;315(8):739–40.
3. Shankar-Hari M, Phillips GS, Levy ML, Seymour CW, Liu VX, Deutschman CS, et al. Developing a new definition and assessing new clinical criteria for septic shock: for the third international consensus definitions for sepsis and septic shock (sepsis-3). JAMA. 2016;315(8):775–87.
4. Singer M, Deutschman CS, Seymour CW, Shankar-Hari M, Annane D, Bauer M, et al. The third international consensus definitions for sepsis and septic shock (sepsis-3). JAMA. 2016;315(8):801–10.
5. Cohen J, Vincent J-L, Adhikari NKJ, Machado FR, Angus DC, Calandra T, et al. Sepsis: a roadmap for future research. Lancet Infect Dis. 2015;15(5):581–614.
6. Adhikari NK, Fowler RA, Bhagwanjee S, Rubenfeld GD. Critical care and the global burden of critical illness in adults. Lancet. 2010;376(9749):1339–46.
7. Hamers L, Kox M, Pickkers P. Sepsis-induced immunoparalysis: mechanisms, markers, and treatment options. Minerva Anestesiol. 2015;81:426–39.
8. Davenport EE, Burnham KL, Radhakrishnan J, Humburg P, Hutton P, Mills TC, Rautanen A, Gordon AC, Garrard C, Hill AVS, Hinds CJ, Knight JC. Genomic landscape of the individual host response and outcomes in severe sepsis. Lancet Respir Med. 2016;4:259–71.
9. Radi R. Peroxynitrite, a stealthy biological oxidant. J Biol Chem. 2013;288:26464–72.
10. Moore JP, Dyson A, Singer M, Fraser J. Microcirculatory dysfunction and resuscitation: why, when, and how. Br J Anaesth. 2015;115(3):366–75.
11. Spronk PE, Zandstra DF, Ince C. Bench-to-bedside review: sepsis is a disease of the microcirculation. Crit Care. 2004;8:462–8.
12. Hernandez G, Bruhn A, Castro R, Regueira T. The holistic view on perfusion monitoring in septic shock. Curr Opin Crit Care. 2012;18(3):280–6.

13. Simmons J, Pittet JF. The coagulopathy of acute sepsis. Curr Opin Anaesthesiol. 2015;28:227–36.
14. Gatewood MO, Wemple M, Greco S, Kritek PA, Durvasula R. A quality improvement project to improve early sepsis care in the emergency department. BMJ Qual Saf. 2015;24:787–95.
15. Jones SL, Ashton CM, Kiehne L, et al. Reductions in sepsis mortality and costs after design and implementation of a nurse-based early recognition and response program. Jt Comm J Qual Patient Saf. 2015;41:483–91.
16. Klein Klouwenberg PM, Cremer OL, van Vught LA, et al. Likelihood of infection in patients with presumed sepsis at the time of intensive care unit admission: a cohort study. Crit Care. 2015;19:319.
17. Contou D, Roux D, Jochmans S, et al. Septic shock with no diagnosis at 24 hours: a pragmatic multicenter prospective cohort study. Crit Care. 2016;20:360.
18. Seymour CW, Liu VX, Iwashyna TJ, et al. Assessment of clinical criteria for sepsis: for the third international consensus definitions for sepsis and septic shock (sepsis-3). JAMA. 2016;315:762–74.
19. Freund Y, Lemachatti N, Krastinova E, et al. Prognostic accuracy of sepsis-3 criteria for in-hospital mortality among patients with suspected infection presenting to the emergency department. JAMA. 2017;317:301–8.
20. Williams JM, Greenslade JH, McKenzie JV, Chu K, Brown AF, Lipman J. Systemic inflammatory response syndrome, quick sequential organ function assessment, and organ dysfunction: insights from a prospective database of ED patients with infection. Chest. 2017;151:586–96.
21. Meurer WJ, Smith BL, Losman ED, et al. Real-time identification of serious infection in geriatric patients using clinical information system surveillance. J Am Geriatr Soc. 2009;57:40–5.
22. Nelson JL, Smith BL, Jared JD, Younger JG. Prospective trial of real-time electronic surveillance to expedite early care of severe sepsis. Ann Emerg Med. 2011;57:500–4.
23. Rivers E, Nguyen B, Havstad S, et al. Early goal-directed therapy in the treatment of severe sepsis and septic shock. N Engl J Med. 2001;345:1368–77.
24. Peake SL, Delaney A, Bailey M, et al. Goal-directed resuscitation for patients with early septic shock. N Engl J Med. 2014;371:1496–506.
25. Yealy DM, Kellum JA, Huang DT, et al. A randomized trial of protocol-based care for early septic shock. N Engl J Med. 2014;370:1683–93.
26. Mouncey PR, Osborn TM, Power GS, et al. Trial of early, goal-directed resuscitation for septic shock. N Engl J Med. 2015;372:1301–11.
27. Rhodes A, Evans LE, Alhazzani W, et al. Surviving sepsis campaign: International guidelines for management of sepsis and septic shock: 2016. Crit Care Med. 2017;45:486–552.
28. Raghunathan K, Bonavia A, Nathanson BH, et al. Association between initial fluid choice and subsequent in-hospital mortality during the resuscitation of adults with septic shock. Anesthesiology. 2015;123:1385–93.
29. Caironi P, Tognoni G, Masson S, et al. Albumin replacement in patients with severe sepsis or septic shock. N Engl J Med. 2014;370:1412–21.
30. Xu JY, Chen QH, Xie JF, et al. Comparison of the effects of albumin and crystalloid on mortality in adult patients with severe sepsis and septic shock: a meta-analysis of randomized clinical trials. Crit Care. 2014;18:702.
31. Jiang L, Jiang S, Zhang M, Zheng Z, Ma Y. Albumin versus other fluids for fluid resuscitation in patients with sepsis: a meta-analysis. PLoS One. 2014;9:e114666.
32. Finfer S, Bellomo R, Boyce N, French J, Myburgh J, Norton R. A comparison of albumin and saline for fluid resuscitation in the intensive care unit. N Engl J Med. 2004;350:2247–56.
33. Perner A, Haase N, Guttormsen AB, et al. Hydroxyethyl starch 130/0.42 versus Ringer's acetate in severe sepsis. N Engl J Med. 2012;367:124–34.
34. Eskesen TG, Wetterslev M, Perner A. Systematic review including re-analyses of 1148 individual data sets of central venous pressure as a predictor of fluid responsiveness. Intensive Care Med. 2016;42:324–32.
35. Cavallaro F, Sandroni C, Marano C, et al. Diagnostic accuracy of passive leg raising for prediction of fluid responsiveness in adults: systematic review and meta-analysis of clinical studies. Intensive Care Med. 2010;36:1475–83.
36. Casserly B, Phillips GS, Schorr C, et al. Lactate measurements in sepsis-induced tissue hypoperfusion: results from the Surviving Sepsis Campaign database. Crit Care Med. 2015;43:567–73.
37. Jansen TC, van Bommel J, Schoonderbeek FJ, et al. Early lactate-guided therapy in intensive care unit patients: a multicenter, open-label, randomized controlled trial. Am J Respir Crit Care Med. 2010;182:752–61.
38. Jones AE, Shapiro NI, Trzeciak S, Arnold RC, Claremont HA, Kline JA. Lactate clearance vs central venous oxygen saturation as goals of early sepsis therapy: a randomized clinical trial. JAMA. 2010;303:739–46.
39. Simpson SQ, Gaines M, Hussein Y, Badgett RG. Early goal-directed therapy for severe sepsis and septic shock: a living systematic review. J Crit Care. 2016;36:43–8.
40. Gu WJ, Zhang Z, Bakker J. Early lactate clearance-guided therapy in patients with sepsis: a meta-analysis with trial sequential analysis of randomized controlled trials. Intensive Care Med. 2015;41:1862–3.
41. Arnold RC, Shapiro NI, Jones AE, et al. Multicenter study of early lactate clearance as a determinant of

survival in patients with presumed sepsis. Shock. 2009;32:35–9.
42. Nguyen HB, Rivers EP, Knoblich BP, et al. Early lactate clearance is associated with improved outcome in severe sepsis and septic shock. Crit Care Med. 2004;32:1637–42.
43. Puskarich MA, Shapiro NI, Massey MJ, Kline JA, Jones AE. Lactate clearance in septic shock is not a surrogate for improved microcirculatory flow. Acad Emerg Med. 2016;23:690–3.
44. Pierrakos C, Vincent JL. Sepsis biomarkers: a review. Crit Care. 2010;14:R15.
45. Simon L, Gauvin F, Amre DK, Saint-Louis P, Lacroix J. Serum procalcitonin and C-reactive protein levels as markers of bacterial infection: a systematic review and meta-analysis. Clin Infect Dis. 2004;39:206–17.
46. Povoa P, Coelho L, Almeida E, et al. C-reactive protein as a marker of infection in critically ill patients. Clin Microbiol Infect. 2005;11:101–8.
47. Schmit X, Vincent JL. The time course of blood C-reactive protein concentrations in relation to the response to initial antimicrobial therapy in patients with sepsis. Infection. 2008;36:213–9.
48. Silvestre J, Povoa P, Coelho L, et al. Is C-reactive protein a good prognostic marker in septic patients? Intensive Care Med. 2009;35:909–13.
49. Wacker C, Prkno A, Brunkhorst FM, Schlattmann P. Procalcitonin as a diagnostic marker for sepsis: a systematic review and meta-analysis. Lancet Infect Dis. 2013;13:426–35.
50. Kopterides P, Siempos II, Tsangaris I, Tsantes A, Armaganidis A. Procalcitonin-guided algorithms of antibiotic therapy in the intensive care unit: a systematic review and meta-analysis of randomized controlled trials. Crit Care Med. 2010;38:2229–41.
51. van der Does Y, Rood PP, Haagsma JA, Patka P, van Gorp EC, Limper M. Procalcitonin-guided therapy for the initiation of antibiotics in the ED: a systematic review. Am J Emerg Med. 2016;34:1286–93.
52. Prkno A, Wacker C, Brunkhorst FM, Schlattmann P. Procalcitonin-guided therapy in intensive care unit patients with severe sepsis and septic shock—a systematic review and meta-analysis. Crit Care. 2013;17:R291.
53. de Jong E, van Oers JA, Beishuizen A, et al. Efficacy and safety of procalcitonin guidance in reducing the duration of antibiotic treatment in critically ill patients: a randomised, controlled, open-label trial. Lancet Infect Dis. 2016;16:819–27.
54. Cardoso T, Carneiro AH, Ribeiro O, Teixeira-Pinto A, Costa-Pereira A. Reducing mortality in severe sepsis with the implementation of a core 6-hour bundle: results from the Portuguese community-acquired sepsis study (SACiUCI study). Crit Care. 2010;14:R83.
55. Ferrer R, Artigas A, Suarez D, et al. Effectiveness of treatments for severe sepsis: a prospective, multicenter, observational study. Am J Respir Crit Care Med. 2009;180:861–6.
56. Weinstein MP, Reller LB, Murphy JR, Lichtenstein KA. The clinical significance of positive blood cultures: a comprehensive analysis of 500 episodes of bacteremia and fungemia in adults. I. Laboratory and epidemiologic observations. Rev Infect Dis. 1983;5:35–53.
57. Baron EJ, Miller JM, Weinstein MP, et al. A guide to utilization of the microbiology laboratory for diagnosis of infectious diseases: 2013 recommendations by the Infectious Diseases Society of America (IDSA) and the American Society for Microbiology (ASM)(a). Clin Infect Dis. 2013;57:e22–e121.
58. Vincent JL, De Backer D. Circulatory shock. N Engl J Med. 2013;369(18):1726–34.
59. Baigorri F, Russell JA. Oxygen delivery in critical illness. Crit Care Clin. 1996;12(4):971–94.
60. Luecke T, Roth H, Herrmann P, Joachim A, Weisser G, Pelosi P, Quintel M. Assessment of cardiac preload and left ventricular function under increasing levels of positive end-expiratory pressure. Intensive Care Med. 2004;30(1):119–26.
61. Marik PE, Monnet X, Teboul JL. Hemodynamic parameters to guide fluid therapy. Ann Intensive Care. 2011;1(1):1.
62. Dellinger RP, Levy MM, Rhodes A, Annane D, Gerlach H, Opal SM, Sevransky JE, Sprung CL, Douglas IS, Jaeschke R, Osborn TM, Nunnally ME, Townsend SR, Reinhart K, Kleinpell RM, Angus DC, Deutschman CS, Machado FR, Rubenfeld GD, Webb SA, Beale RJ, Vincent JL, Moreno R, Surviving Sepsis Campaign Guidelines Committee including the Pediatric Subgroup. Surviving sepsis campaign: international guidelines for management of severe sepsis and septic shock: 2012. Crit Care Med. 2013;41(2):580–637.
63. Osman D, Ridel C, Ray P, Monnet X, Anguel N, Richard C, Teboul JL. Cardiac filling pressures are not appropriate to predict hemodynamic response to volume challenge. Crit Care Med. 2007;35(1):64–8.
64. Marik PE, Cavallazzi R. Does the central venous pressure predict fluid responsiveness? An updated meta-analysis and a plea for some common sense. Crit Care Med. 2013;41(7):1774–81.
65. Prekker ME, Scott NL, Hart D, Sprenkle MD, Leatherman JW. Point-of-care ultrasound to estimate central venous pressure: a comparison of three techniques. Crit Care Med. 2013;41(3):833–41.
66. Muller L, Bobbia X, Toumi M, Louart G, Molinari N, Ragonnet B, Quintard H, Leone M, Zoric L, Lefrant JY, AzuRea Group. Respiratory variations of inferior vena cava diameter to predict fluid responsiveness in spontaneously breathing patients with acute circulatory failure: need for a cautious use. Crit Care. 2012;16(5):R188.
67. Wang CH, Hsieh WH, Chou HC, Huang YS, Shen JH, Yeo YH, Chang HE, Chen SC, Lee

CC. Liberal versus restricted fluid resuscitation strategies in trauma patients: a systematic review and meta-analysis of randomized controlled trials and observational studies. Crit Care Med. 2014;42(4):954–61.
68. Jozwiak M, Silva S, Persichini R, Anguel N, Osman D, Richard C, Teboul JL, Monnet X. Extravascular lung water is an independent prognostic factor in patients with acute respiratory distress syndrome. Crit Care Med. 2013;41(2):472–80.
69. Micek ST, McEvoy C, McKenzie M, Hampton N, Doherty JA, Kollef MH. Fluid balance and cardiac function in septic shock as predictors of hospital mortality. Crit Care. 2013;17(5):R246.
70. Mackenzie DC. Noble VE2. Assessing volume status and fluid responsiveness in the emergency department. Clin Exp Emerg Med. 2014;1(2):67–77.
71. Marik PE, Cavallazzi R, Vasu T, Hirani A. Dynamic changes in arterial waveform derived variables and fluid responsiveness in mechanically ventilated patients: a systematic review of the literature. Crit Care Med. 2009;37(9):2642–7.
72. Guinot PG, de Broca B, Abou Arab O, Diouf M, Badoux L, Bernard E, Lorne E, Dupont H. Ability of stroke volume variation measured by oesophageal Doppler monitoring to predict fluid responsiveness during surgery. Br J Anaesth. 2013;110(1):28–33.
73. De Backer D, Heenen S, Piagnerelli M, Koch M, Vincent JL. Pulse pressure variations to predict fluid responsiveness: influence of tidal volume. Intensive Care Med. 2005;31(4):517–23.
74. Soubrier S, Saulnier F, Hubert H, Delour P, Lenci H, Onimus T, Nseir S, Durocher A. Can dynamic indicators help the prediction of fluid responsiveness in spontaneously breathing critically ill patients? Intensive Care Med. 2007;33(7):1117–24.
75. Biais M, de Courson H, Lanchon R, Pereira B, Bardonneau G, Griton M, Sesay M, Nouette-Gaulain K. Mini-fluid challenge of 100 ml of crystalloid predicts fluid responsiveness in the operating room. Anesthesiology. 2017;127(3):450–6.
76. Guinot PG, Bernard E, Defrancq F, Petiot S, Majoub Y, Dupont H, Lorne E. Mini-fluid challenge predicts fluid responsiveness during spontaneous breathing under spinal anaesthesia: An observational study. Eur J Anaesthesiol. 2015;32(9):645–9.
77. Leisman DE, Goldman C, Doerfler ME, Masick KD, Dries S, Hamilton E, Narasimhan M, Zaidi G, D'Amore JA, D'Angelo JK. Patterns and outcomes associated with timeliness of initial crystalloid resuscitation in a prospective sepsis and septic shock cohort. Crit Care Med. 2017;45(10):1596–606. https://doi.org/10.1097/CCM.0000000000002574.
78. Leisman D, Wie B, Doerfler M, Bianculli A, Ward MF, Akerman M, D'Angelo JK, Zemmel D'Amore JA. Association of fluid resuscitation initiation within 30 minutes of severe sepsis and septic shock recognition with reduced mortality and length of stay. Ann Emerg Med. 2016;68(3):298–311.
79. Sperry JL, Minei JP, Frankel HL, West MA, Harbrecht BG, Moore EE, Maier RV, Nirula R. Early use of vasopressors after injury: caution before constriction. J Trauma. 2008;64(1):9–14.
80. Mouncey PR, Osborn TM, Power GS, Harrison DA, Sadique MZ, Grieve RD, Jahan R, Harvey SE, Bell D, Bion JF, Coats TJ, Singer M, Young JD, Rowan KM. ProMISe Trial Investigators. Trial of early, goal-directed resuscitation for septic shock. N Engl J Med. 2015;372(14):1301–11.
81. Weiskopf RB, Viele MK, Feiner J, Kelley S, Lieberman J, Noorani M, Leung JM, Fisher DM, Murray WR, Toy P, Moore MA. Human cardiovascular and metabolic response to acute, severe isovolemic anemia. JAMA. 1998;279(3):217–21.
82. Holst LB, Haase N, Wetterslev J, Wernerman J, Guttormsen AB, Karlsson S, Johansson PI, Aneman A, Vang ML, Winding R, Nebrich L, Nibro HL, Rasmussen BS, Lauridsen JR, Nielsen JS, Oldner A, Pettilä V, Cronhjort MB, Andersen LH, Pedersen UG, Reiter N, Wiis J, White JO, Russell L, Thornberg KJ, Hjortrup PB, Müller RG, Møller MH, Steensen M, Tjäder I, Kilsand K, Odeberg-Wernerman S, Sjøbø B, Bundgaard H, Thyø MA, Lodahl D, Mærkedahl R, Albeck C, Illum D, Kruse M, Winkel P, Perner A, TRISS Trial Group; Scandinavian Critical Care Trials Group. Lower versus higher hemoglobin threshold for transfusion in septic shock. N Engl J Med. 2014;371(15):1381–91.
83. Hébert PC, Yetisir E, Martin C, Blajchman MA, Wells G, Marshall J, Tweeddale M, Pagliarello G, Schweitzer I, Transfusion Requirements in Critical Care Investigators for the Canadian Critical Care Trials Group. Is a low transfusion threshold safe in critically ill patients with cardiovascular diseases? Crit Care Med. 2001;29(2):227–34.
84. Surviving Sepsis Campaign Bundles-Revised 4/2015 by the SSC Executive Committee. http://www.survivingsepsis.org/SiteCollectionDocuments/SSC_Bundle.pdf.
85. Myburgh JA, Finfer S, Bellomo R, Billot L, Cass A, Gattas D, Glass P, Lipman J, Liu B, McArthur C, McGuinness S, Rajbhandari D, Taylor CB, Webb SA, CHEST Investigators; Australian and New Zealand Intensive Care Society Clinical Trials Group. Hydroxyethyl starch or saline for fluid resuscitation in intensive care. N Engl J Med. 2012;367(20):1901–11.
86. Yunos NM, Bellomo R, Hegarty C, Story D, Ho L, Bailey M. Association between a chloride-liberal vs chloride-restrictive intravenous fluid administration strategy and kidney injury in critically ill adults. JAMA. 2012;308(15):1566–72.
87. Rochwerg B, Alhazzani W, Sindi A, Heels-Ansdell D, Thabane L, Fox-Robichaud A, Mbuagbaw L, Szczeklik W, Alshamsi F, Altayyar S, Ip WC, Li G,

Wang M, Wludarczyk A, Zhou Q, Guyatt GH, Cook DJ, Jaeschke R, Annane D, Fluids in Sepsis and Septic Shock Group. Fluid resuscitation in sepsis: a systematic review and network meta-analysis. Ann Intern Med. 2014;161(5):347–55.
88. Acheampong A, Vincent JL. A positive fluid balance is an independent prognostic factor in patients with sepsis. Crit Care. 2015;19:251.
89. Mitchell KH, Carlbom D, Caldwell E, Leary PJ, Himmelfarb J, Hough CL. Volume overload: prevalence, risk factors, and functional outcome in survivors of septic shock. Ann Am Thorac Soc. 2015;12(12):1837–44.
90. Delaney AP, Dan A, McCaffrey J, Finfer S. The role of albumin as a resuscitation fluid for patients with sepsis: a systematic review and meta-analysis. Crit Care Med. 2011;39(2):386–91.
91. Zhang Z, Chen K. Vasoactive agents for the treatment of sepsis. Ann Transl Med. 2016;4(17):333.
92. De Backer D, Biston P, Devriendt J, Madl C, Chochrad D, Aldecoa C, Brasseur A, Defrance P, Gottignies P, Vincent JL. SOAP II Investigators. Comparison of dopamine and norepinephrine in the treatment of shock. N Engl J Med. 2010;362(9):779–89.
93. Marik PE, Mohedin M. The contrasting effects of dopamine and norepinephrine on systemic and splanchnic oxygen utilization in hyperdynamic sepsis. JAMA. 1994;272(17):1354–7.
94. Patel GP, Grahe JS, Sperry M, Singla S, Elpern E, Lateef O, Balk RA. Efficacy and safety of dopamine versus norepinephrine in the management of septic shock. Shock. 2010;33(4):375–80.
95. Russell JA, Walley KR, Singer J, Gordon AC, Hébert PC, Cooper DJ, Holmes CL, Mehta S, Granton JT, Storms MM, Cook DJ, Presneill JJ, Ayers D, VASST Investigators. Vasopressin versus norepinephrine infusion in patients with septic shock. N Engl J Med. 2008;358(9):877–87.
96. Gordon AC, Mason AJ, Thirunavukkarasu N, Perkins GD, Cecconi M, Cepkova M, Pogson DG, Aya HD, Anjum A, Frazier GJ, Santhakumaran S, Ashby D, Brett SJ, VANISH Investigators. Effect of early vasopressin vs norepinephrine on kidney failure in patients with septic shock: the vanish randomized clinical trial. JAMA. 2016;316(5):509–18.
97. Landry DW, Levin HR, Gallant EM, Ashton RC Jr, Seo S, D'Alessandro D, Oz MC, Oliver JA. Vasopressin deficiency contributes to the vasodilation of septic shock. Circulation. 1997;95(5):1122–5.
98. Ferrer R, Martin-Loeches I, Phillips G, Osborn TM, Townsend S, Dellinger RP, Artigas A, Schorr C, Levy MM. Empiric antibiotic treatment reduces mortality in severe sepsis and septic shock from the first hour: results from a guideline-based performance improvement program. Crit Care Med. 2014;42(8):1749–55.
99. Gaieski DF, Mikkelsen ME, Band RA, Pines JM, Massone R, Furia FF, Shofer FS, Goyal M. Impact of time to antibiotics on survival in patients with severe sepsis or septic shock in whom early goal-directed therapy was initiated in the emergency department. Crit Care Med. 2010;38(4):1045–53.
100. Funk DJ, Kumar A. Antimicrobial therapy for life-threatening infections: speed is life. Crit Care Clin. 2011;27(1):53–76.
101. NICE-SUGAR Study Investigators, Finfer S, Chittock DR, Su SY, Blair D, Foster D, Dhingra V, Bellomo R, Cook D, Dodek P, Henderson WR, Hébert PC, Heritier S, Heyland DK, McArthur C, McDonald E, Mitchell I, Myburgh JA, Norton R, Potter J, Robinson BG, Ronco JJ. Intensive versus conventional glucose control in critically ill patients. N Engl J Med. 2009;360(13):1283–97.
102. Keh D, Trips E, Marx G, Wirtz SP, Abduljawwad E, Bercker S, Bogatsch H, Briegel J, Engel C, Gerlach H, Goldmann A, Kuhn SO, Hüter L, Meier-Hellmann A, Nierhaus A, Kluge S, Lehmke J, Loeffler M, Oppert M, Resener K, Schädler D, Schuerholz T, Simon P, Weiler N, Weyland A, Reinhart K, Brunkhorst FM, SepNet–Critical Care Trials Group. Effect of hydrocortisone on development of shock among patients with severe sepsis: the HYPRESS randomized clinical trial. JAMA. 2016;316(17):1775–85.
103. Sprung CL, Annane D, Keh D, Moreno R, Singer M, Freivogel K, Weiss YG, Benbenishty J, Kalenka A, Forst H, Laterre PF, Reinhart K, Cuthbertson BH, Payen D, Briegel J, CORTICUS Study Group. Hydrocortisone therapy for patients with septic shock. N Engl J Med. 2008;358(2):111–24.
104. Annane D, Sébille V, Charpentier C, Bollaert PE, François B, Korach JM, Capellier G, Cohen Y, Azoulay E, Troché G, Chaumet-Riffaud P, Bellissant E. Effect of treatment with low doses of hydrocortisone and fludrocortisone on mortality in patients with septic shock. JAMA. 2002;288(7):862–71.
105. Weber-Carstens S, Deja M, Bercker S, Dimroth A, Ahlers O, Kaisers U, Keh D. Impact of bolus application of low-dose hydrocortisone on glycemic control in septic shock patients. Intensive Care Med. 2007;33(4):730–3.
106. Mestas J, Hughes CC. Of mice and not men: differences between mouse and human immunology. J Immunol. 2004;172(5):2731–8.
107. Dyson A, Singer M. Animal models of sepsis: why does preclinical efficacy fail to translate to the clinical setting? Crit Care Med. 2009;37(1 Suppl):S30–7.
108. Fink MP, Warren HS. Strategies to improve drug development for sepsis. Nat Rev Drug Discov. 2014;13(10):741–58.
109. Minneci PC, Deans KJ, Eichacker PQ, Natanson C. The effects of steroids during sepsis depend on dose and severity of illness: an updated meta-analysis. Clin Microbiol Infect. 2009;15(4):308–18.

110. Berry SM, Connor JT, Lewis RJ. The platform trial: an efficient strategy for evaluating multiple treatments. JAMA. 2015;313(16):1619–20.
111. Gattinoni L, Brazzi L, Pelosi P, Latini R, Tognoni G, Pesenti A, et al. A trial of goal-oriented hemodynamic therapy in critically ill patients. SvO2 Collaborative Group. N Engl J Med. 1995;333(16):1025–32.
112. Raghunathan K, Shaw A, Nathanson B, Sturmer T, Brookhart A, Stefan MS, et al. Association between the choice of IV crystalloid and in-hospital mortality among critically ill adults with sepsis*. Crit Care Med. 2014;42(7):1585–91.
113. Zampieri FG, Ranzani OT, Azevedo LC, Martins ID, Kellum JA, Liborio AB. Lactated ringer is associated with reduced mortality and less acute kidney injury in critically ill patients: a retrospective cohort analysis. Crit Care Med. 2016;44(12):2163–70.
114. Patel A, Laffan MA, Waheed U, Brett SJ. Randomised trials of human albumin for adults with sepsis: systematic review and meta-analysis with trial sequential analysis of all-cause mortality. BMJ. 2014;349:g4561.
115. Monnet X, Teboul JL. Assessment of volume responsiveness during mechanical ventilation: recent advances. Crit Care. 2013;17(2):217.
116. Asfar P, Meziani F, Hamel JF, Grelon F, Megarbane B, Anguel N, et al. High versus low blood-pressure target in patients with septic shock. N Engl J Med. 2014;370(17):1583–93.
117. Seymour CW, Gesten F, Prescott HC, Friedrich ME, Iwashyna TJ, Phillips GS, et al. Time to treatment and mortality during mandated emergency care for sepsis. N Engl J Med. 2017;376(23):2235–44.
118. Ziegler R, Johnscher I, Martus P, Lenhardt D, Just HM. Controlled clinical laboratory comparison of two supplemented aerobic and anaerobic media used in automated blood culture systems to detect bloodstream infections. J Clin Microbiol. 1998;36(3):657–61.
119. Bochud PY, Bonten M, Marchetti O, Calandra T. Antimicrobial therapy for patients with severe sepsis and septic shock: an evidence-based review. Crit Care Med. 2004;32(11 Suppl):S495–512.
120. Bouadma L, Luyt CE, Tubach F, Cracco C, Alvarez A, Schwebel C, et al. Use of procalcitonin to reduce patients' exposure to antibiotics in intensive care units (PRORATA trial): a multicentre randomised controlled trial. Lancet. 2010;375(9713):463–74.
121. Jensen JU, Hein L, Lundgren B, Bestle MH, Mohr TT, Andersen MH, et al. Procalcitonin-guided interventions against infections to increase early appropriate antibiotics and improve survival in the intensive care unit: a randomized trial. Crit Care Med. 2011;39(9):2048–58.
122. Layios N, Lambermont B, Canivet JL, Morimont P, Preiser JC, Garweg C, et al. Procalcitonin usefulness for the initiation of antibiotic treatment in intensive care unit patients. Crit Care Med. 2012;40(8):2304–9.
123. Calfee CS, Delucchi K, Parsons PE, Thompson BT, Ware LB, Matthay MA, et al. Subphenotypes in acute respiratory distress syndrome: latent class analysis of data from two randomised controlled trials. Lancet Respir Med. 2014;2(8):611–20.
124. Famous KR, Delucchi K, Ware LB, Kangelaris KN, Liu KD, Thompson BT, et al. Acute respiratory distress syndrome subphenotypes respond differently to randomized fluid management strategy. Am J Respir Crit Care Med. 2017;195(3):331–8.
125. Delmas A, Leone M, Rousseau S, Albanese J, Martin C. Clinical review: Vasopressin and terlipressin in septic shock patients. Crit Care. 2005;9(2):212–22.
126. Asfar P, Russell JA, Tuckermann J, Radermacher P. Selepressin in septic shock: a step toward decatecholaminization? Crit Care Med. 2016;44(1):234–6.
127. Khanna A, English SW, Wang XS, Ham K, Tumlin J, Szerlip H, et al. Angiotensin II for the treatment of vasodilatory shock. N Engl J Med. 2017;377(5):419–30.
128. Cordemans C, De Laet I, Van Regenmortel N, Schoonheydt K, Dits H, Huber W, et al. Fluid management in critically ill patients: the role of extravascular lung water, abdominal hypertension, capillary leak, and fluid balance. Ann Intensive Care. 2012;2(Suppl 1 Diagnosis and management of intra-abdominal hyperten):S1.
129. Han S, Lee SJ, Kim KE, Lee HS, Oh N, Park I, et al. Amelioration of sepsis by TIE2 activation-induced vascular protection. Sci Transl Med. 2016;8(335):335ra55.
130. Opal SM, Laterre PF, Francois B, LaRosa SP, Angus DC, Mira JP, et al. Effect of eritoran, an antagonist of MD2-TLR4, on mortality in patients with severe sepsis: the ACCESS randomized trial. JAMA. 2013;309(11):1154–62.
131. Ranieri VM, Thompson BT, Barie PS, Dhainaut JF, Douglas IS, Finfer S, et al. Drotrecogin alfa (activated) in adults with septic shock. N Engl J Med. 2012;366(22):2055–64.
132. Meisel C, Schefold JC, Pschowski R, Baumann T, Hetzger K, Gregor J, et al. Granulocyte-macrophage colony-stimulating factor to reverse sepsis-associated immunosuppression: a double-blind, randomized, placebo-controlled multicenter trial. Am J Respir Crit Care Med. 2009;180(7):640–8.
133. Fink MP. Cytopathic hypoxia. Mitochondrial dysfunction as mechanism contributing to organ dysfunction in sepsis. Crit Care Clin. 2001; 17(1):219–37.
134. Schmidt H, Muller-Werdan U, Hoffmann T, Francis DP, Piepoli MF, Rauchhaus M, et al. Autonomic dysfunction predicts mortality in patients with multiple organ dysfunction syndrome of different age groups. Crit Care Med. 2005;33(9):1994–2002.

135. Morelli A, Ertmer C, Westphal M, Rehberg S, Kampmeier T, Ligges S, et al. Effect of heart rate control with esmolol on hemodynamic and clinical outcomes in patients with septic shock: a randomized clinical trial. JAMA. 2013;310(16):1683–91.
136. Tyndall A, Pistoia V. Mesenchymal stem cells combat sepsis. Nat Med. 2009;15(1):18–20.
137. Pandharipande PP, Girard TD, Jackson JC, Morandi A, Thompson JL, Pun BT, et al. Long-term cognitive impairment after critical illness. N Engl J Med. 2013;369(14):1306–16.
138. Heming N, Mazeraud A, Verdonk F, Bozza FA, Chretien F, Sharshar T. Neuroanatomy of sepsis-associated encephalopathy. Crit Care. 2017;21(1):65.

Anaphylaxis: Early Recognition and Management

6

Won Young Kim

6.1 Introduction

Anaphylaxis is a serious systemic allergic reaction with a sudden onset after exposure to an offending agent [1]. Signs and symptoms can range from relatively mild to life threatening. About 2% of the population suffers from anaphylaxis during their lifetime; common causes are food, medications, and insect stings [2]. Recently the incidence of anaphylaxis is increasing in many countries; the prevention and treatment of anaphylaxis is an important clinical emergency which all healthcare professionals should be able to recognize and manage. Despite the release of a number of guidelines and updated practice on the management of anaphylaxis, there are identified gaps in knowledge and practice as well as barriers to care in emergency department (ED) [3]. Many of the gaps in the treatment of anaphylaxis included the lack of a practical definition of anaphylaxis as it related to physician.

The most well-known consensus clinical definition of anaphylaxis was proposed by Second National Institute of Allergy and Infection Disease/Food Allergy and Anaphylaxis Network Symposium (NIAID/FAAN) in 2005 [4]. The World Allergy Organization (WAO) Guidelines for the assessment and management of anaphylaxis (subsequently referred to as the Guidelines) were published on 3 March 2011 [1]. Recently, the European Academy of Allergy and Clinical Immunology (EAACI) released the EAACI Guidelines for Food Allergy to provide evidence-based recommendations for the recognition, risk assessment, and management of patients who are at risk of experiencing anaphylaxis [5].

The cornerstone of anaphylaxis management is the use of epinephrine as a first-line treatment while reserving H1-antihistamines and corticosteroids as second-line agents. Useful second-line interventions may include removing the trigger where possible, calling for help, correct positioning of the patient, high-flow oxygen, intravenous fluids, and inhaled short-acting bronchodilators. Biphasic anaphylactic reactions have been reported to develop in up to 20% of reactions although the evidence for this is of low quality. In general, patients with moderate respiratory or cardiovascular events should be monitored for at least 4–6 h and, if necessary, up to 24 h [6, 7]. In this chapter, we review and summarize the early recognition and management of anaphylaxis.

6.2 Pathophysiology

Anaphylaxis is an acute, potentially lethal, multisystem syndrome resulting from the sudden release of mast cell-, basophil-, and macrophage-derived mediators into the circulation [8]. The typical

W. Y. Kim
Department of Emergency Medicine, University of Ulsan College of Medicine, Asan Medical Center, Seoul, South Korea

G. J. Suh (ed.), *Essentials of Shock Management*, https://doi.org/10.1007/978-981-10-5406-8_6

pathophysiology of anaphylaxis involves immunoglobulin E (IgE). The term of anaphylactoid reaction has been used to describe IgE-independent events, although the two reactions are often clinically indistinguishable. The WAO dedicated to allergy and clinical immunology has proposed discarding this nomenclature [4]. The WAO categorizes anaphylaxis as either immunologic or non-immunologic. Immunologic anaphylaxis includes both IgE-mediated and IgG-mediated reactions, and immune complex/complement-mediated mechanisms [1]. Non-immunologic anaphylaxis is caused by agents or events that induce sudden, massive mast cell or basophil degranulation, without the involvement of antibodies [1]. Triger factors vary by region, age, and season. Food is the most common cause but drug and insect infestations are relatively common in older adults.

6.3 Initial Approach and Diagnosis

Traditionally, anaphylaxis was defined as based on mechanistically IgE-dependent reaction or on clinical reactions that range from urticarial to life threatening such as hypotension or shock. However, this definition is not useful for non-allergists. Anaphylaxis is defined as a "severe, life-threatening systemic hypersensitivity reaction"; this is characterized by being rapid in onset with life-threatening airway, breathing, or circulatory problems and is usually, although not always, associated with skin and mucosal changes [1]. This definition suggests that the diagnosis of anaphylaxis is based on clinical symptoms and signs. The current clinical criteria for diagnosing anaphylaxis are published in NIAID/FAAN second symposium and WAO guidelines (Table 6.1). These widely accepted criteria significantly improve the identification of anaphylaxis and can lead to rapid management.

The first step of the diagnosis of anaphylaxis should be based on the detailed history of clinical symptoms and all substances such as food, exercise, and medications exposed within a few hours before symptoms appear. Symptoms and signs usually occur within 2 h of exposure to the allergen, usually within 30 min for food allergy and even faster with parenteral medication or insect stings [5]. In a large case series of fatal anaphylaxis, the median time from symptoms to

Table 6.1 Definition of anaphylaxis [1, 4]

Anaphylaxis is highly likely when any one of the following three criteria is fulfilled:	
Criteria 1	
Acute onset of an illness (minutes to several hours) with involvement of the skin, mucosal tissue, or both (e.g., pruritus or flushing, swollen lips–tongue–uvula) And at least ONE of the following	(a) Respiratory compromise (e.g., dyspnea, wheeze–bronchospasm, stridor, reduced PEF, hypoxemia) (b) Reduced BP or associated symptoms of end-organ dysfunction (e.g., hypotonia [collapse], syncope, incontinence)
Or Criteria 2	
Two or more of the following that occur rapidly after exposure to a likely allergen for that patient (minutes to several hours):	(a) Involvement of the skin–mucosal tissue (e.g., generalized hives, itch-flush, swollen lips–tongue–uvula (b) Respiratory compromise (e.g., dyspnea, wheeze–bronchospasm, stridor, hypoxemia) (c) Reduced BP or associated symptoms (e.g., hypotonia [collapse], syncope, incontinence) (d) Persistent gastrointestinal symptoms (e.g., crampy abdominal pain, vomiting)
Or Criteria 3	
Reduced BP after exposure to known allergen for that patient (minutes to several hours):	(a) Infants and children: low systolic BP (age specific) or >30% decrease in systolic BP[a] (b) Adults: systolic BP of <90 mmHg or >30% decrease from that person's baseline

[a]Low systolic blood pressure for children is defined as <70 mmHg from 1 month to 1 year, less than (70 mmHg + [29 age]) from 1 to 10 years and <90 mmHg from 11 to 17 years

arrest has been reported as 30, 15, and 5 min for food, insect venom, and parenteral medication, respectively [9].

The clinical manifestations of anaphylaxis depend on the organ systems involved. Multiple symptoms occurring in at least two or more organs such as mucous membrane including skin, respiratory system, cardiovascular system, nervous system, and gastrointestinal system are typical. Thus, the second step of the diagnosis of anaphylaxis is detecting involved organ system. It should be noted that there are five types of involved system, but consensus definition of anaphylaxis classifies into four systems by combining cardiovascular and nervous system (Table 6.1). Among the symptoms of anaphylaxis, cutaneous manifestations occur in most cases. In a recent study describing a cohort of 340 adult patients with anaphylaxis, the skin and mucocutaneous such as pruritus or flushing and swollen lips–tongue–uvula were the most frequently affected organs (86%), followed by respiratory symptoms (68%), cardiovascular and neurologic symptoms (55%), and gastrointestinal symptoms (35%) [10]. However, the symptoms of anaphylaxis differ from person to person for the same cause. Attention should be paid that a patient can have anaphylaxis without shock. Moreover, the progression of anaphylaxis from itching to death is unpredictable. Even when the initial symptoms are mild, there is significant potential for rapid progression to a severe reaction. Thus physician should be familiar with the three diagnostic criteria of anaphylaxis and patients with these symptoms meeting the criteria should be treated as soon as possible.

Blood tests are not necessary for the diagnosis of anaphylaxis. However, measuring serum tryptase and histamine may help to distinguish other diseases with similar symptoms. Blood samples for measurement of tryptase levels are optimally obtained 15 min to 3 h after symptom onset. When the diagnosis is uncertain, serum tryptase greater than 2.0 μg/L at the time of symptom onset 1–2 h often supports the clinical diagnosis of anaphylaxis [11]. However, in anaphylaxis due to food or anaphylaxis without hypotension, tryptase may show normal results because basophils are more involved than mast cells [12].

6.4 Management

Anaphylaxis is a medical emergency. Prompt assessment and management are critically important. In this section of the Guidelines, we discuss a systematic approach to the basic initial management of anaphylaxis, emphasizing the primary role of epinephrine in treatment. It is also important to note that any delay in appropriate treatment increases the potential for morbidity and mortality [7, 13].

6.4.1 Airway Management

Although treatment of choice is epinephrine for anaphylaxis management, the immediate steps involve a rapid assessment of the patient's airway. Intubation should be performed in patients with developing airway compromise and early intubation should be considered if significant edema of tongue, uvula, or voice alteration has developed, especially in patients with short time since the exposure.

6.4.2 Epinephrine

The first-line use of epinephrine is the standard of care for anaphylaxis and is a clear directive in all gridlines [1, 14]. Delaying administration of epinephrine has been associated with increased reaction severity, increased morbidity, a greater likelihood of biphasic reactions, and an increased risk of fatality even in some cases in which the initial symptoms were mild [15–17]. However, recent analysis with nation-wide data on the management of anaphylaxis found that there is a distinct discrepancy between current guidelines and their implementation; for example only 13.0% received epinephrine [18]. To improve the treatment of anaphylaxis, they strongly recommend revision of medical education and practical training.

6.4.2.1 Mechanisms of Action

Epinephrine is lifesaving because of its alpha-1 adrenergic vasoconstrictor effects in most body organ systems (skeletal muscle is an important exception) and its ability to prevent and relieve airway obstruction caused by mucosal edema, and to prevent and relieve hypotension and shock [1, 15, 19]. Other relevant properties in anaphylaxis include its beta-1 adrenergic agonist inotropic and chronotropic properties leading to an increase in the force and rate of cardiac contractions, and its beta-2 adrenergic agonist properties such as decreased mediator release, bronchodilation, and relief of urticaria [20, 21].

6.4.2.2 Route and Dose

Epinephrine should be injected by the intramuscular route in the mid-anterolateral thigh as soon as anaphylaxis is diagnosed or strongly suspected, in a dose of 0.01 mg/kg of a 1:1000 (1 mg/mL) solution, to a maximum of 0.5 mg in adults (0.3 mg in children) [4, 6, 20, 22, 23]. Depending on the severity of the episode and the response to the initial injection, the dose can be repeated every 5–15 min, as needed. Most patients respond to one or two doses of epinephrine injected intramuscularly promptly; however, more than two doses are occasionally required. Failure to inject it promptly is potentially associated with fatality.

Epinephrine can be given by slow intravenous infusion with diluted solution 1:10,000 (0.1 mg/mL), ideally with the dose titrated according to noninvasive continuous monitoring of cardiac rate and function [22]. For example, if shock is imminent or has already developed or cardiac arrest is impending, an intravenous bolus dose of epinephrine is indicated; however, in other anaphylaxis scenarios, this route of administration should be avoided [20].

6.4.2.3 Adverse Effect

Transient pharmacologic effects after a recommended dose of epinephrine by any route of administration include pallor, tremor, anxiety, palpitations, dizziness, and headache [15, 19, 20]. These symptoms indicate that a therapeutic dose has been given. Serious adverse effects such as ventricular arrhythmias, hypertensive crisis, and pulmonary edema potentially occur after an overdose of epinephrine by any route of administration. Typically, they are reported after intravenous epinephrine dosing [9, 20]. Moreover intravenous epinephrine injection can lead to dosing error and epinephrine overdose [24]. Physician should be aware that there are no absolute contraindications to the use of epinephrine for anaphylaxis and serious adverse effects are very rare when epinephrine is administrated at the appropriate intramuscular doses for anaphylaxis.

6.4.3 Intravenous Fluids

Patients with anaphylaxis should not suddenly sit, stand, or be placed in the upright position because massive fluid shifts can occur in anaphylaxis. All patients with orthostasis, hypotension, or incomplete response to epinephrine should receive large-volume fluid resuscitation with isotonic saline or normal saline. The rate of administration should be titrated according to the blood pressure, cardiac rate and function, and urine output. All patients receiving such treatment should be monitored for volume overload. Normotensive patients should receive normal saline to maintain venous access in case their status deteriorates.

6.4.4 Second-Line Pharmacologic Treatment

6.4.4.1 H1-Antihistamine

H1-antihistamines relieve itching, flushing, urticaria, angioedema, and nasal and eye symptoms; however, they should not be substituted for epinephrine because they are not lifesaving; that is, they do not prevent or relieve upper airway obstruction, hypotension, or shock [4, 20, 22, 23]. Moreover it does not inhibit mediator release from mast cells and basophils and rapid intravenous administration may increase hypotension. Some guidelines do not recommend H1-antihistamine treatment in anaphylaxis, citing lack of supporting evidence from randomized controlled trials that meet current standards [25]. Current systematic review reported that no high-quality evidence was found to support the use of H1-antihistamines in the treatment of anaphylaxis [26].

6.4.4.2 H2-Antihistamine

An H2-antihistamine, administered concurrently with an H1-antihistamine, potentially contributes to decrease in flushing, headache, and other symptoms; however, H2-antihistamines are recommended in only a few anaphylaxis guidelines [22, 27]. Moreover, rapid intravenous administration of cimetidine has been reported to increase hypotension [22] and anaphylaxis to ranitidine has been reported [28].

6.4.4.3 Glucocorticoids

Glucocorticoids switch off transcription of a multitude of activated genes that encode proinflammatory proteins. Extrapolating from their use in acute asthma, the onset of action of systemic glucocorticoids takes several hours [29]. Although they potentially relieve protracted anaphylaxis symptoms and prevent biphasic anaphylaxis [20, 22], these effects have never been proven. Therefore, glucocorticoid is not lifesaving in initial hours of an anaphylactic episode. Current systematic review failed to identify any evidence to confirm the effectiveness of glucocorticoids in the treatment of anaphylaxis, and raised concerns that they are often inappropriately used as first-line medications in place of epinephrine [30].

6.4.4.4 Bronchodilators

Selective beta-2 adrenergic agonists such as salbutamol (albuterol) are sometimes given in anaphylaxis as additional treatment for wheezing, coughing, and shortness of breath not relieved by epinephrine. Although this is helpful for lower respiratory tract symptoms, these medications should not be substituted for epinephrine because they have minimal alpha-1 adrenergic agonist vasoconstrictor effects and do not prevent or relieve laryngeal edema and upper airway obstruction, hypotension, or shock [20] (Table 6.2).

Table 6.2 Initial management and medications of anaphylaxis [20]

Basic initial management
1. Remove exposure to the trigger, if possible For example, discontinue an intravenous diagnostic or therapeutic agent that seems to be triggering symptoms 2. Assess circulation, airway, breathing, mental status, skin, and body weight 3. Call for help (resuscitation team in hospital or emergency medical services in community setting), if available 4. Inject epinephrine intramuscularly in the mid-anterolateral aspect of the thigh, 0.01 mg/kg of a 1:1000 (1 mg/mL) solution, to a maximum of 0.5 mg (adult) or 0.3 mg (childe); record the time of the dose and repeat it in 5–15 min, if needed; most patients respond to one or two doses 5. Place patient on the back, or in a position of comfort if there is respiratory distress and/or vomiting; elevate the lower extremities; fatality can occur within seconds if a patient stands or sits suddenly 6. Give high-flow supplemental oxygen (6–8 L/min) by face mask or oropharyngeal airway 7. Establish intravenous access with wide-bore cannula. When indicated, give 1–2 L of 0.9% (isotonic) saline rapidly (e.g., 5–10 mL/kg in the first 5–10 min to an adult, or 10 mL/kg to a child) 8. When indicated at any time, prepare to initiate cardiopulmonary resuscitation with continuous chest compressions
Medications
1. First-line (priority) medication – Epinephrine 1:1000 (1 mg/mL) intramuscular injection 0.01 mg/kg, to a maximum of 0.5 mg (adult), 0.3 mg (child) 2. Second-line medications – H1-antihistamine for intravenous infusion For example chlorpheniramine 10 mg (adult), 2.5–5 mg (child) or diphenhydramine 25–50 mg (adult) (1 mg/kg, maximum 50 mg [child]) – ß2-adrenergic agonist For example salbutamol (albuterol) solution, 2.5 mg/3 mL or 5 mg/3 mL (adult), (2.5 mg/3 mL [child]) given by nebulizer and face mask – Glucocorticoid for intravenous infusion For example hydrocortisone 200 mg (adult), maximum 100 mg (child); or methylprednisolone 50–100 mg (adult); 1 mg/kg, maximum 50 mg (child) – H2-antihistamine for intravenous infusion For example, ranitidine 50 mg (adult) or 1 mg/kg, maximum 50 mg (child)

6.4.5 Management of Refractory Anaphylaxis

A minority of patients do not respond to timely, basic initial anaphylaxis treatment with epinephrine by intramuscular injection, supplemental oxygen, intravenous fluid resuscitation, and second-line medications. In these refractory anaphylaxis patients with shock, no clear superiority of dopamine, dobutamine, norepinephrine, phenylephrine, or vasopressin (either added to epinephrine alone or compared with one another) has been demonstrated in clinical trials. Physicians suspect patients taking a beta-adrenergic blocker or other medications that interfere with epinephrine effect. Glucagon, a polpypeptide with non-catecholamine-dependent inotropic and chronotropic cardiac effects, is sometimes needed in patients taking a beta-adrenergic blocker who have hypotension and bradycardia and who do not respond optimally to epinephrine [31].

Patients suffering from refractory anaphylaxis have been resuscitated with extracorporeal membrane oxygenation (ECMO) or operative cardiopulmonary bypass. ECMO is becoming increasingly available in ED and should be considered in patients unresponsive to complete resuscitative efforts in institutions with experience in this technology. The decision to initiate ECMO should be considered early in patients unresponsive to traditional resuscitative measures, before irreversible ischemic acidosis develops.

6.5 Disposition

The duration of monitoring of the developing biphasic anaphylaxis after initial treatment varies from patient to patient. In general, patients with moderate respiratory or cardiovascular events should be monitored for at least 4 h, and if indicated for 8–10 h or longer, and patients with severe or protracted anaphylaxis might require monitoring and interventions for days. For the biphasic anaphylaxis, timely epinephrine administration appears to have a role, but the role of steroids has been called into question and is an opportunity for future investigation.

6.5.1 Biphasic Reaction

6.5.1.1 Incidence and Risk Factor

A biphasic anaphylactic reaction was first described in 1984 and was defined as the recurrence of symptoms after complete resolution of initial anaphylactic without re-exposure to the trigger [32]. The reported incidence rate varies from 3 to 20% depending on the study population, and recent systemic review of 4162 patients showed a 4.6% rate of biphasic reaction [32]. It may occur from 1 to 72 h after the first anaphylactic reaction. Guidelines about optimal duration of observation vary considerably in their recommendations: the United States recommend 6 h of observation after the initial anaphylactic episode due to the risk of a biphasic reaction [7], and Europe recommends up to 24 h of observation [6]. Identifying patients who are most likely to benefit from a longer period of observation is important. However, risk factors for developing a biphasic anaphylaxis have not been well studied due to the uncommon occurrence. In observational studies with 415 anaphylaxis patients from Korea, history of drug anaphylaxis (odds ratio 14.3, 95% CI 2.4–85.8) was a contributing factor to the development of the biphasic reaction [33]. A recent systemic review found that initial presentation with hypotension (odds ratio 2.18, 95% CI 1.1–4.2) was associated with the development of the biphasic reaction and anaphylaxis due to food was associated with decreased risk (odds ratio 0.62, 95% CI 0.4–0.94) [32]. In addition, the single pediatric study showed that biphasic reactions seem to be associated with the severity of the initial anaphylactic reactions [34]. More studies regarding the identification of anaphylaxis patients at higher risk for biphasic anaphylaxis may be warranted.

6.5.1.2 Prevention

Steroid use and early epinephrine administration have been theorized to decrease biphasic anaphylaxis [35]. However, contemporary studies have failed to find compelling evidence of a protective effect of steroids for preventing biphasic reactions [33, 36]. Recent study of corticosteroid use for the patients with allergy or anaphylaxis did not decrease ED return visits within 7 days [37].

Delayed epinephrine treatment for the initial reaction has been reported as an associated factor with a biphasic reaction [38]. A recent observational study reported that a subgroup of patients who had delays in their initial epinephrine administration were more likely to develop biphasic reactions [34]. The role of other allergy medications in the prevention of biphasic anaphylaxis is not well studied.

6.5.2 Epinephrine Auto-Injector

In patients with anaphylaxis, it can be recurred due to re-exposure to the substance or stimulant. Therefore, patients with anaphylaxis, even after initial successful treatment, should be educated to avoid antigen and usage of epinephrine auto-injector. Patients should be advised that they have experienced a potentially life-threatening medical emergency ("killer allergy"), and that if their symptoms recur within the next 72 h they should inject epinephrine and call emergency medical services or be taken to the nearest emergency facility [20].

6.6 Future

Inappropriate treatment of anaphylaxis can be caused by failure of early recognition. We believed that the early recognition with three clinical diagnostic criteria, use of epinephrine as soon as possible, and appropriate discharge plans were the most critical recommendations for ED health professionals. At a time when anaphylaxis is increasing, physicians also should recognize that anaphylaxis may not appear life threatening and that the patients may present without respiratory or cardiovascular symptoms. For the biphasic anaphylaxis which is a debating issue, timely epinephrine administration appears to have a role, but the role of steroids has been called into question and is an opportunity for future investigation. Moreover, studies regarding the identification of anaphylaxis patients at higher risk for biphasic anaphylaxis may be warranted.

References

1. Simons FE, Ardusso LR, Bilo MB, El-Gamal YM, Ledford DK, Ring J, et al. World Allergy Organization anaphylaxis guidelines: summary. J Allergy Clin Immunol. 2011a;127(3):587-93.e1-22. https://doi.org/10.1016/j.jaci.2011.01.038.
2. Yu JE, Lin RY. The epidemiology of anaphylaxis. Clin Rev Allergy Immunol. 2015; https://doi.org/10.1007/s12016-015-8503-x.
3. Russell WS, Farrar JR, Nowak R, Hays DP, Schmitz N, Wood J, et al. Evaluating the management of anaphylaxis in US emergency departments: guidelines vs. practice. World J Emerg Med. 2013;4(2):98–106. https://doi.org/10.5847/wjem.j.1920-8642.2013.02.003.
4. Sampson HA, Munoz-Furlong A, Campbell RL, Adkinson NF Jr, Bock SA, Branum A, et al. Second symposium on the definition and management of anaphylaxis: summary report—Second National Institute of Allergy and Infectious Disease/Food Allergy and Anaphylaxis Network symposium. J Allergy Clin Immunol. 2006a;117(2):391–7. https://doi.org/10.1016/j.jaci.2005.12.1303.
5. Muraro A, Roberts G, Worm M, Bilo MB, Brockow K, Fernandez Rivas M, et al. Anaphylaxis: guidelines from the European Academy of Allergy and Clinical Immunology. Allergy. 2014;69(8):1026–45. https://doi.org/10.1111/all.12437.
6. Muraro A, Roberts G, Clark A, Eigenmann PA, Halken S, Lack G, et al. The management of anaphylaxis in childhood: position paper of the European academy of allergology and clinical immunology. Allergy. 2007;62(8):857–71. https://doi.org/10.1111/j.1398-9995.2007.01421.x.
7. Sampson HA, Munoz-Furlong A, Campbell RL, Adkinson NF Jr, Bock SA, Branum A, et al. Second symposium on the definition and management of anaphylaxis: summary report—second National Institute of Allergy and Infectious Disease/Food Allergy and Anaphylaxis Network symposium. Ann Emerg Med. 2006b;47(4):373–80. https://doi.org/10.1016/j.annemergmed.2006.01.018.
8. Johansson SG, Bieber T, Dahl R, Friedmann PS, Lanier BQ, Lockey RF, et al. Revised nomenclature for allergy for global use: report of the nomenclature review committee of the World Allergy Organization, october 2003. J Allergy Clin Immunol. 2004;113(5):832–6. https://doi.org/10.1016/j.jaci.2003.12.591.

9. Pumphrey RS. Lessons for management of anaphylaxis from a study of fatal reactions. Clin Exp Allergy. 2000;30(8):1144–50.
10. Ko BS, Kim JY, Seo DW, Kim WY, Lee JH, Sheikh A, et al. Should adrenaline be used in patients with hemodynamically stable anaphylaxis? Incident case control study nested within a retrospective cohort study. Sci Rep. 2016;6:20168. https://doi.org/10.1038/srep20168.
11. Sala-Cunill A, Cardona V, Labrador-Horrillo M, Luengo O, Esteso O, Garriga T, et al. Usefulness and limitations of sequential serum tryptase for the diagnosis of anaphylaxis in 102 patients. Int Arch Allergy Immunol. 2013;160(2):192–9. https://doi.org/10.1159/000339749.
12. Caughey GH. Tryptase genetics and anaphylaxis. J Allergy Clin Immunol. 2006;117(6):1411–4. https://doi.org/10.1016/j.jaci.2006.02.026.
13. Sampson HA, Munoz-Furlong A, Bock SA, Schmitt C, Bass R, Chowdhury BA, et al. Symposium on the definition and management of anaphylaxis: summary report. J Allergy Clin Immunol. 2005;115(3):584–91. https://doi.org/10.1016/j.jaci.2005.01.009.
14. Boyce JA, Assa'ad A, Burks AW, Jones SM, Sampson HA, Wood RA, et al. Guidelines for the diagnosis and management of food allergy in the United States: report of the NIAID-sponsored expert panel. J Allergy Clin Immunol. 2010a;126(6 Suppl):S1–58. https://doi.org/10.1016/j.jaci.2010.10.007.
15. Kemp SF, Lockey RF, Simons FE. Epinephrine: the drug of choice for anaphylaxis. A statement of the World Allergy Organization. Allergy. 2008;63(8):1061–70. https://doi.org/10.1111/j.1398-9995.2008.01733.x.
16. Nowak R, Farrar JR, Brenner BE, Lewis L, Silverman RA, Emerman C, et al. Customizing anaphylaxis guidelines for emergency medicine. J Emerg Med. 2013;45(2):299–306. https://doi.org/10.1016/j.jemermed.2013.01.018.
17. Simons FE. Anaphylaxis. J Allergy Clin Immunol. 2010;125(2 Suppl 2):S161–81. https://doi.org/10.1016/j.jaci.2009.12.981.
18. Grabenhenrich L, Hompes S, Gough H, Rueff F, Scherer K, Pfohler C, et al. Implementation of anaphylaxis management guidelines: a register-based study. PLoS One. 2012;7(5):e35778. https://doi.org/10.1371/journal.pone.0035778.
19. Simons KJ, Simons FE. Epinephrine and its use in anaphylaxis: current issues. Curr Opin Allergy Clin Immunol. 2010;10(4):354–61. https://doi.org/10.1097/ACI.0b013e32833bc670.
20. Simons FE, Ardusso LR, Bilo MB, El-Gamal YM, Ledford DK, Ring J, et al. World allergy organization guidelines for the assessment and management of anaphylaxis. World Allerg Organ J. 2011b;4(2):13–37. https://doi.org/10.1097/WOX.0b013e318211496c.
21. Smith PL, Kagey-Sobotka A, Bleecker ER, Traystman R, Kaplan AP, Gralnick H, et al. Physiologic manifestations of human anaphylaxis. J Clin Investig. 1980;66(5):1072–80. https://doi.org/10.1172/jci109936.
22. Lieberman P, Nicklas RA, Oppenheimer J, Kemp SF, Lang DM, Bernstein DI, et al. The diagnosis and management of anaphylaxis practice parameter: 2010 update. J Allergy Clin Immunol. 2010;126(3):477-80.e1-42. https://doi.org/10.1016/j.jaci.2010.06.022.
23. Soar J, Pumphrey R, Cant A, Clarke S, Corbett A, Dawson P, et al. Emergency treatment of anaphylactic reactions—guidelines for healthcare providers. Resuscitation. 2008;77(2):157–69. https://doi.org/10.1016/j.resuscitation.2008.02.001.
24. Kanwar M, Irvin CB, Frank JJ, Weber K, Rosman H. Confusion about epinephrine dosing leading to iatrogenic overdose: a life-threatening problem with a potential solution. Ann Emerg Med. 2010;55(4):341–4. https://doi.org/10.1016/j.annemergmed.2009.11.008.
25. Brown SG, Mullins RJ, Gold MS. Anaphylaxis: diagnosis and management. Med J Aust. 2006;185(5):283–9.
26. Sheikh A, Ten Broek V, Brown SG, Simons FE. H1-antihistamines for the treatment of anaphylaxis: Cochrane systematic review. Allergy. 2007;62(8):830–7. https://doi.org/10.1111/j.1398-9995.2007.01435.x.
27. Boyce JA, Assa'ad A, Burks AW, Jones SM, Sampson HA, Wood RA, et al. Guidelines for the diagnosis and management of food allergy in the United States: summary of the NIAID-sponsored expert panel report. J Allergy Clin Immunol. 2010b;126(6):1105–18. https://doi.org/10.1016/j.jaci.2010.10.008.
28. Foti C, Cassano N, Panebianco R, Calogiuri GF, Vena GA. Hypersensitivity reaction to ranitidine: description of a case and review of the literature. Immunopharmacol Immunotoxicol. 2009;31(3):414–6. https://doi.org/10.1080/08923970902739078.
29. Rowe BH, Spooner C, Ducharme FM, Bretzlaff JA, Bota GW. Early emergency department treatment of acute asthma with systemic corticosteroids. Cochrane Database Syst Rev. 2001;(1):Cd002178. https://doi.org/10.1002/14651858.cd002178.
30. Choo KJ, Simons E, Sheikh A. Glucocorticoids for the treatment of anaphylaxis: cochrane systematic review. Allergy. 2010;65(10):1205–11. https://doi.org/10.1111/j.1398-9995.2010.02424.x.
31. Thomas M, Crawford I. Best evidence topic report. Glucagon infusion in refractory anaphylactic shock in patients on beta-blockers. Emerg Med J. 2005;22(4):272–3. https://doi.org/10.1136/emj.2005.023507.
32. Lee S, Bellolio MF, Hess EP, Erwin P, Murad MH, Campbell RL. Time of onset and predictors of biphasic anaphylactic reactions: a systematic review and meta-analysis. J Allergy Clin Immunol Pract. 2015;3(3):408-16.e1-2. https://doi.org/10.1016/j.jaip.2014.12.010.

33. Ko BS, Kim WY, Ryoo SM, Ahn S, Sohn CH, Seo DW, et al. Biphasic reactions in patients with anaphylaxis treated with corticosteroids. Ann Allergy Asthma Immunol. 2015;115(4):312–6. https://doi.org/10.1016/j.anai.2015.07.015.
34. Alqurashi W, Stiell I, Chan K, Neto G, Alsadoon A, Wells G. Epidemiology and clinical predictors of biphasic reactions in children with anaphylaxis. Ann Allergy Asthma Immunol. 2015;115(3):217-23.e2. https://doi.org/10.1016/j.anai.2015.05.013.
35. Lieberman P. Biphasic anaphylactic reactions. Ann Allergy Asthma Immunol. 2005;95(3):217–26; quiz 26, 58. https://doi.org/10.1016/s1081-1206(10)61217-3.
36. Rohacek M, Edenhofer H, Bircher A, Bingisser R. Biphasic anaphylactic reactions: occurrence and mortality. Allergy. 2014;69(6):791–7. https://doi.org/10.1111/all.12404.
37. Grunau BE, Wiens MO, Rowe BH, McKay R, Li J, Yi TW, et al. Emergency department corticosteroid use for allergy or anaphylaxis is not associated with decreased relapses. Ann Emerg Med. 2015;66(4):381–9. https://doi.org/10.1016/j.annemergmed.2015.03.003.
38. Smit DV, Cameron PA, Rainer TH. Anaphylaxis presentations to an emergency department in Hong Kong: incidence and predictors of biphasic reactions. J Emerg Med. 2005;28(4):381–8. https://doi.org/10.1016/j.jemermed.2004.11.028.

Part III

Scenario-Based Approach

Scenario-Based Approach

7

Gil Joon Suh, Jae Hyuk Lee, Kyung Su Kim,
Hui Jai Lee, and Joonghee Kim

7.1 Hypovolemic Shock Due to Multiple Trauma

A 32-year-old man came to the emergency department (ED) for multiple trauma. He was found in a parking lot and was suspected to be fallen down from a nearby building. He was transferred to the ED by an emergency medical system with a cervical collar in place and strapped to a backboard. He was confused and anxious, and could not remember the situation at the time of injury, but he was able to follow commands at the ED arrival. His initial vital signs were 55/45 mmHg–124 bpm–22 cpm–32.6 °C with SpO2 at 96%. He was anxious

G. J. Suh (✉)
Department of Emergency Medicine,
Seoul National University College of Medicine,
Seoul, South Korea
e-mail: suhgil@snu.ac.kr

J. H. Lee · J. Kim
Department of Emergency Medicine,
Seoul National University Bundang Hospital,
Gyeonggi-do, South Korea

K. S. Kim
Department of Emergency Medicine,
Seoul National University Hospital,
Seoul, South Korea

H. J. Lee
Department of Emergency Medicine,
Seoul Nation University—Seoul Metropolitan
Government Boramae Medical Center,
Seoul, South Korea
e-mail: emdrlee@snu.ac.kr

Q. Describe initial evaluation steps for this patient.

A. Initial assessment of a multiple trauma patient (primary survey) must be performed promptly. The Advanced Trauma Life Support (ATLS) guideline provides an organized approach focused on identifying life-threatening conditions. It consisted of the following components (ABCDEs). Any problems identified should be managed immediately before moving on to the next step:

1. Airway maintenance with cervical spine protection:
   - A. Ask the patient simple question.
   - B. Observe the patient for signs of respiratory difficulty.
   - C. Inspect oropharyngeal cavity.
   - D. Assess the neck for injuries.
   - E. Protect (immobilize) the C-spine.
2. Breathing and ventilation:
   - A. Assess the adequacy of oxygenation and ventilation.
   - B. Look for chest injuries.
3. Circulation with hemorrhage control:
   - A. Check for bleeding and hemodynamic abnormalities.
   - B. Secure IV lines and control bleeding.
   - C. Reversal of anticoagulation.

G. J. Suh (ed.), *Essentials of Shock Management*, https://doi.org/10.1007/978-981-10-5406-8_7

4. Disability:
   A. Check for neurologic abnormalities.
5. Exposure/environmental control:
   A. Undress the patient and examine the entire body.
   B. Avoid hypothermia.

Q. Which category of hemorrhagic shock does the patient belongs to? What is your initial volume resuscitation strategy?

A. Initial blood pressure of the patient was 55/45 mmHg and pulse rate was 124/min, and he was anxious and confused. Therefore, it is class III hemorrhagic shock. Therefore, the patient needs blood transfusion as well as crystalloid infusion. The colloid solutions (dextran or albumin) have not been demonstrated to be superior to crystalloids. If there is no evidence of significant brain injury, the target systolic blood pressure should be 80–90 mmHg. However, higher blood pressure is recommended in patients with traumatic brain injury (see page 25).

and confused. His right limbs and pelvis had open wounds and deformities. He was suspicious for multiple facial bone fractures, including mandible fracture with oral bleeding and dislodged teeth.

After administration of 2 L of 0.9% saline solution, his blood pressure was increased to 95/60 mmHg with heart rate of 110/min. However, after 10 min his blood pressure dropped to 60/40 mmHg again. During the fluid resuscitation, limb splint and pelvic immobilization were applied to control possible hemorrhages from fractures in the limbs and pelvis. There was involuntary muscle guarding in right upper quadrant area of the abdomen and the focused assessment with sonography in trauma (FAST) identified free fluid in the Morrison's pouch and pneumothorax in the right thorax (Figs. 7.1 and 7.2).

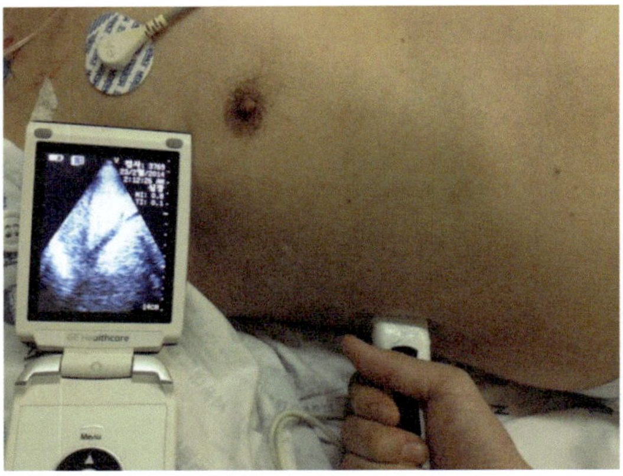

Fig. 7.1 Fast examination of the patient. Fluid collection in the Morrison's pouch (arrow) was observed

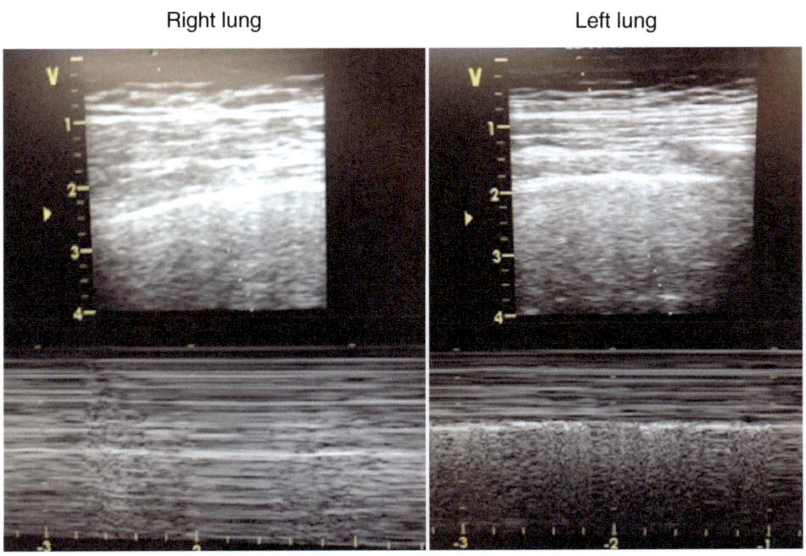

Fig. 7.2 Lung sonography findings of the patient. Right lung scan (left image) shows "barcode sign" while left lung scan (right image) shows "sandy beach sign" in M-mode

Arterial blood gas analysis			CBC			Chemistry			Cardiac enzyme			Coagulation panel			Urinalysis		
pH	7.36		WBC	22,130	/μL	Na	139.5	mmol/L	CK	650	ng/mL	PT (INR)	1.22	INR	WBC	1–4	/HPF
pCO2	37.9	mmHg	Hb	13.3	g/dL	K	3.7	mmol/L	CK-MB	11.2	ng/mL	aPTT	26.5	Seconds	RBC	5–9	/HPF
pO2	174.5	mmHg	Hct	38.8	%	Cl	105.8	mmol/L	TnI	0.3	pg/mL	D-dimer	35.2	μg/mL	Albumin	Negative	
HCO3-	20.9	mmol/L	Platelet	283,000	/μL	TCO2	20.4	mmol/L							Nitrite	Negative	
Base excess	−2.4	mmol/L				BUN	13	mg/dL							Bacteria	Negative	
Lactate	NA	mmol/L				Cr	1.18	mg/dL									
						AST	148	IU/L									
						ALT	87	IU/L									
						T.bil	1	mg/dL									
						ALP	68	IU/L									
						T.prot.	6.4	g/dL									
						Albumin	4	g/dL									

Q. His initial hemoglobin and hematocrit were 13.3 g/dL and 38.8%. Do you think they can represent the severity of acute blood loss?

A. Low hemoglobin and hematocrit are markers of severe bleeding, but normal hemoglobin and hematocrit may not reflect the volume of bleeding. Therefore, serial measurement combined with clinical and imaging study could help assess the volume of bleeding.

Meanwhile, the initial blood test results came out.

Initial chest X-ray was taken during resuscitation. Multiple rib fractures in the right thorax and hemopneumothorax in the right lung field were observed. Right-tube thoracostomy was performed (Fig. 7.3).

In CT angiography, liver laceration in S5 and 6 with active bleeding was identified (Fig. 7.4).

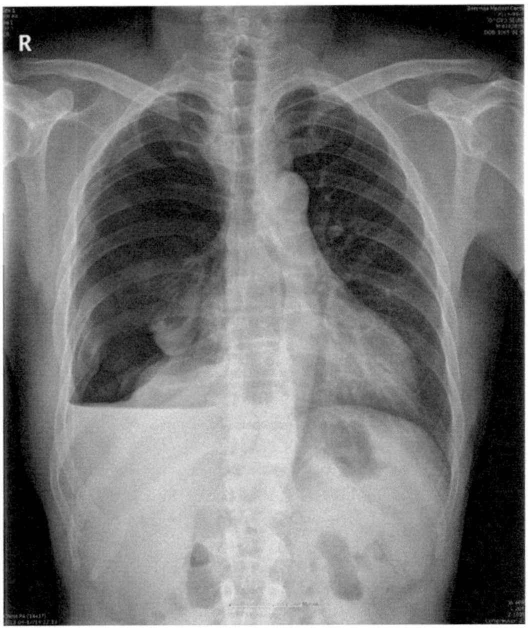

Fig. 7.3 Chest X-ray of the patient showing multiple rib fractures and hemopneumothorax in the right thorax

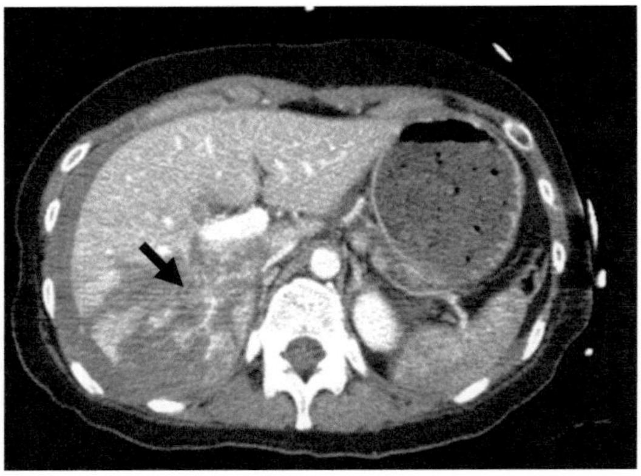

Fig. 7.4 An abdominal CT angiography imaging showing liver laceration in segments 5 and 6 with active contrast vacation (arrow)

Q. Despite blood transfusion, the patient's blood pressure decreased and his pulse rate increased again after the CT angiography. What should you do next?

A. It is **suspected** that this patient has still ongoing bleeding. It is important to control bleeding immediately. Recently, angiographic embolization is gaining popularity for controlling arterial bleeding in patients with hemorrhage shock. However, it should not delay consultation for surgical bleeding control. In this case, surgical consultation for bleeding control should be done first. If surgical treatment is not possible, multidisciplinary approach should be considered, such as angiographic embolization (see page 29).

7.1.1 Progression

The patient was transferred to the operating room for surgical control of arterial bleeding in the liver. After surgical treatment, he was admitted to the intensive care unit for close observation. Then, after 2 weeks of intensive care unit treatment, he was recovered and discharged home.

7.1.2 Summary

This is a case of hemorrhagic shock in multiple trauma. The estimated blood loss of this patient was about 30–40% according to hemorrhagic shock classification. He was initially resuscitated with crystalloid. However, the hemodynamic response was transient. Thus, immediate blood transfusion was performed. To assess bleeding focus, FAST exam was performed and it revealed intra-abdominal free fluid. For further assessment of bleeding focus, CT angiography was performed. The main bleeding focus was found to be liver laceration on CT angiography. The patient was moved to operating room for surgical bleeding control.

7.2 A Hemorrhagic Shock Case Treated with REBOA

A 46-year-old male without underlying disease came to the emergency department (ED) for falling from seventh floor of apartment for purpose of suicide. His initial vital signs were 110/60 mmHg–102 bpm–20 cpm–36.4 °C with saturation at 95%. He was slightly drowsy but able to move arms by following doctor's instructions. He complained of pain in pelvis and back and deformity in right forearm at the arrival time, but there was no definite open wound on his body.

Q. What is the first step of assessing the patient?

A. Primary survey (ABCDEs) should be accompanied by appropriate resuscitations:

1. Airway maintenance with cervical spine protection.
2. Breathing and ventilation.
3. Circulation with hemorrhage control.
4. Disability: neurologic status.
5. Exposure/environmental control (see page 93).

In primary survey, there was no tender point in face, cervical spine, and upper trunk and his respiration was stable. No definite open wound or external bleeding was observed. He could move both hands and feet but could not flex both hip joints because of pain.

FAST was performed to assess injury of internal organs and bleeding during initial evaluation and it showed that there was no definite fluid collection at pericardium and intra-abdominal spaces.

In secondary survey, he looked a little pale. Lung sound was clear in both lung fields and there was no definite painful area during palpating chest wall. When his abdomen was palpated, he complained of pain at the right side of abdomen. Multiple bruises and swellings were shown at his back and buttocks after changing position with logrolling manners. He could not flex both legs because of severe pelvic pain, but could move both knees and ankles. Deformity of right forearm was also observed.

During the secondary survey, he became confused and his skin was pale and wet. His blood pressure dropped (VS: 56/36 mmHg–108 bpm–23 cpm–36.0 °C).

Q. According to the Advanced Trauma Life Support (ATLS) guidelines, in which class is this patient included?

A. He had tachycardia, hypotension, and altered mentality (confusion). These indicate that the patient is in class III hemorrhagic shock. Estimated volume of blood loss is 1500–2000 mL in 70 kg male (see page 21).

Fluid resuscitation with 0.9% saline solution of 2000 mL was performed and endotracheal intubation was performed to protect airway. However, his blood pressure was still low at 65/40 mmHg and heart rate was 128 bpm. A repeated FAST was performed to find delayed internal hemorrhage which showed free fluids in the Morrison's pouch and pelvic cavity (Fig. 7.5).

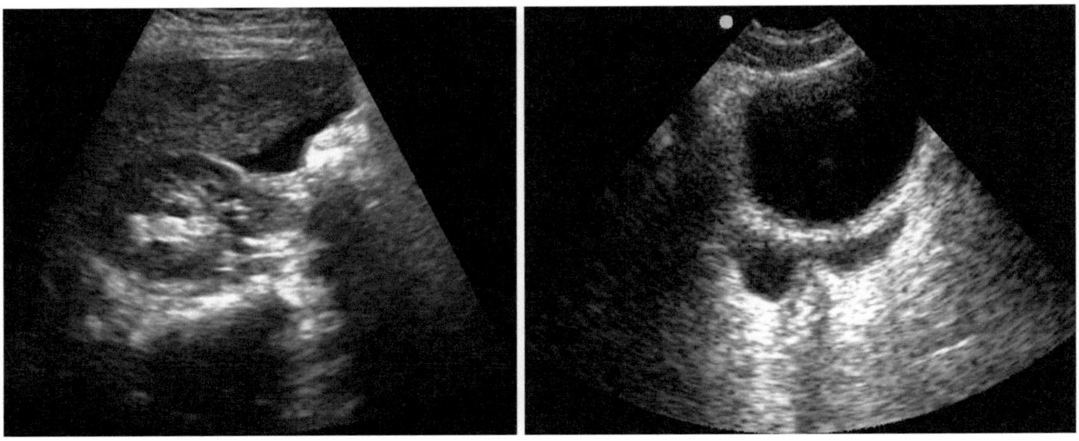

Fig. 7.5 Free fluid in the Morrison's pouch and pelvic cavity

Q. Does he need massive transfusion? If so, what is your rationale for massive transfusion?

A. He requires massive transfusion according to ABC score. The ABC score has four parameters including penetrating torso injury, systolic blood pressure ≤90 mmHg, heart rate ≥120 bpm, and positive focused assessment with sonography for trauma (FAST). His ABC score was three and massive transfusion would be necessary for this patient (see page 27).

Q. What is your initial plan for transfusion and how much for initial transfusion?

A. Resuscitation with FFP, platelets, and RBCs at 1:1:1 unit ratios has been recommended for massive transfusion for trauma patients. If you are going to transfuse the patient with 1:1:1 ratio, minimal 4 units of p-RBC, 4 units of FFP, and 4 units of platelet are necessary (see page 27).

Q. Which antifibrinolytic agent can be used for the patients who need massive transfusion?

A. Tranexamic acid and the recommended dose is a loading dose of 1 g over 10 min, followed by infusion of 1 g over 8 h (see pages 27–28).

Pelvic X-rays and CT scan were performed. Multiple pelvic bone fractures and right retroperitoneal hematoma were identified (Fig. 7.6).

Massive transfusion protocol was initiated, but his blood pressure remained low at 85/48 mmHg with a heart rate of 107 bpm. Norepinephrine was started and titrated up to 40 μg/min. Meanwhile his initial laboratory report came out (Fig. 7.7).

Arterial blood gas analysis			CBC			Chemistry			Cardiac enzyme			Coagulation panel			Urinalysis		
pH	7.306		WBC	18,700	/μL	Na	138	mmol/L	CK	24.4	ng/mL	PT (INR)	1.98	INR	WBC	<1	/HPF
pCO2	30.3	mmHg	Hb	6.8	g/dL	K	3	mmol/L	CK-MB	1.73	ng/mL	aPTT	50.3	Seconds	RBC	<1	/HPF
pO2	79.9	mmHg	Hct	20.1	%	Cl	105	mmol/L	TnI	NA	pg/mL	D-dimer	>20	μg/mL	Albumin	Negative	
HCO3-	17.3	mmol/L	Platelet	129,000	/μL	TCO2	19	mmol/L							Nitrite	Negative	
Base excess	−4.2	mmol/L				BUN	19	mg/dL							Bacteria	Negative	
Latate	5.8	mmol/L				Cr	1.81	mg/dL									
						AST	82	IU/L									
						ALT	39	IU/L									
						T.bil	0.6	mg/dL									
						ALP	50	IU/L									
						T.prot.	3.5	g/dL									
						Albumin	4	g/dL									

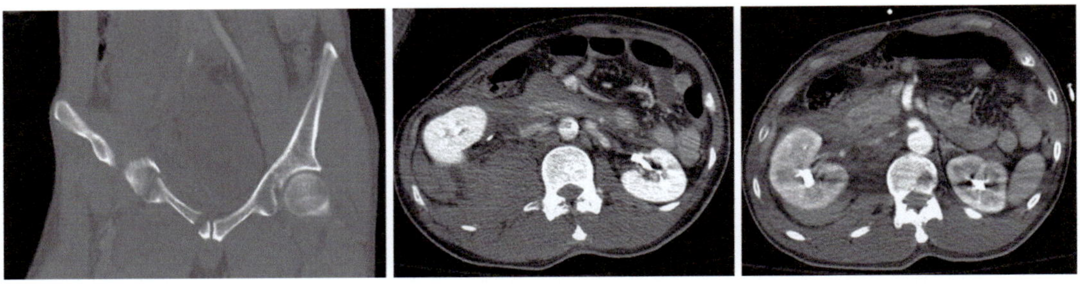

Fig. 7.6 Abdominopelvic CT showing multiple pelvic fractures and hematoma in the right retroperitoneum

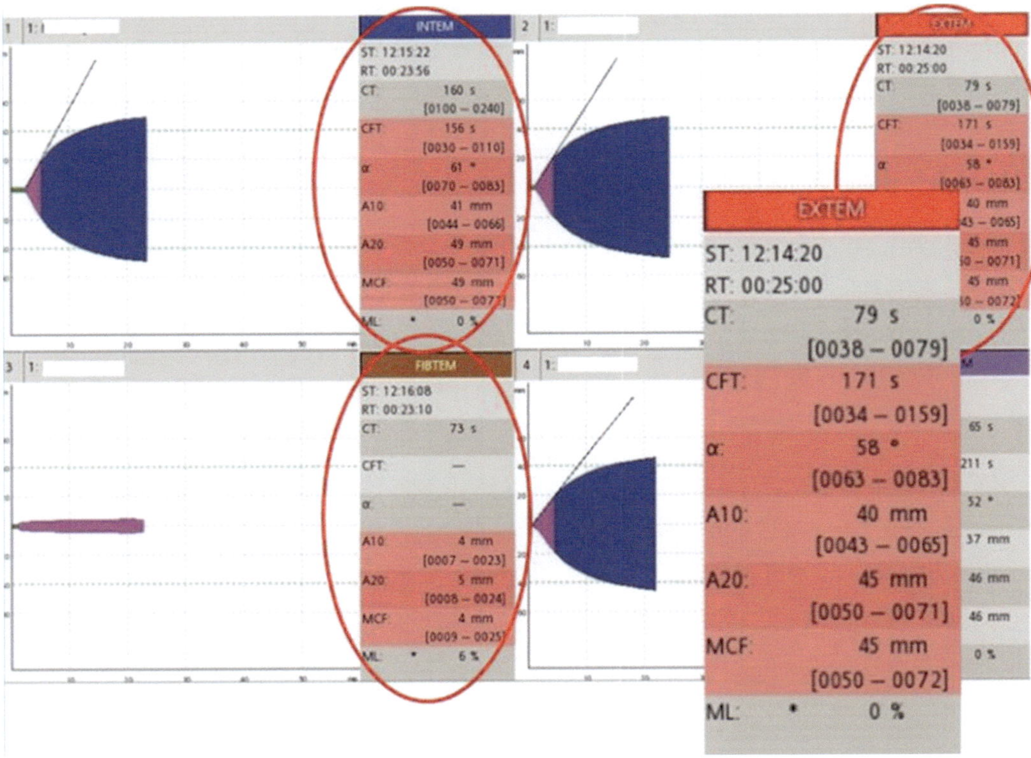

Fig. 7.7 ROTEM results of the patient. $A10_{EX}$ and $A10_{FIB}$ were decreased to 40 mm and 4 mm, respectively. $A10_{EX}$, amplitude 10 min after coagulation time in EXTEM; $A10_{FIB}$, amplitude 10 min after coagulation time in FIBTEM

Q. What is your strategy for assessment and management of trauma-induced coagulopathy?

A. Thromboelastography (TEG) and rotational thromboelastometry (ROTEM) can be used to monitor trauma-induced coagulopathy rapidly at bedside. These examinations show important variables such as clotting time, clot formation/kinetics, clot strengthening, amplitude/maximal firmness, and lysis, by analyzing clot formation kinetics (see pages 23–24).

Q. Which management is needed to correct the value of ROTEM?

A. Amplitude 10 min after coagulation time in EXTEM ($A10_{EX}$) was decreased to 40 mm, and amplitude 10 min after coagulation time in FIBTEM ($A10_{FIB}$) was decreased to 4 mm, so he needed to get fibrinogen concentrates or cryoprecipitate till $A10_{FIB}$ reached 12 mm. Coagulation time in INTEM (CT_{IN}) and coagulation time in EXTEM (CT_{EX}) were within normal limit and correction is not needed.

Despite the massive transfusion, the patient was still in hypotension with BP at 70/45 mmHg. While waiting for angiographic intervention for embolization, the treating ED physicians decided to use resuscitative endovascular balloon occlusion of the aorta (REBOA) to control active bleeding. The device was introduced via femoral artery under the fluoroscopic guidance and the blood pressure increased rapidly to 134/51 mmHg after inflation of its balloon. Infusion of norepinephrine was titrated down to 4 μg/min.

He was moved to angiography room. Hypervascular staining was supplied by engorged both internal iliac arteries with vascular spasm of distal branches in aortography and both internal iliac arteriogrphy. Embolization of both internal iliac arteries using glue and gelfoam was done. The REBOA was removed from patient after balloon deflation (Fig. 7.8).

His vital sign became stable after embolization. Additional radiography showed fracture of ulnar proximal shaft with dislocation of radius head in right arm. He was admitted to surgical intensive care unit for 10 days. He got open reduction and external screw fixation of multiple pelvic bone fracture, right radius, and ulnar fractures at the hospital day 9. Neuropsychiatric consultation was done after recovery of mental status and he was diagnosed with schizophrenia with major depressive disorder. He was discharged and transferred to local hospital for rehabilitation at the hospital day 33.

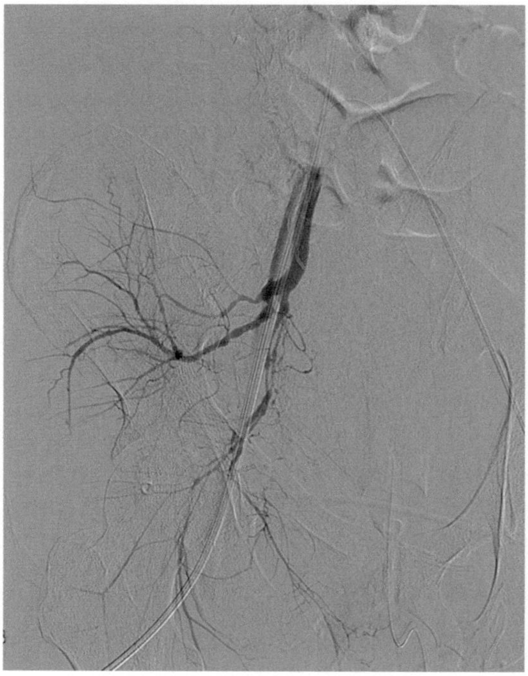

Fig. 7.8 Embolization of both internal iliac arteries using glue and gelfoam

7.2.1 Summary

This was a case of uncontrolled hemorrhagic shock in multiple trauma. In this case, initial resuscitation for refractory hemorrhagic shock was not possible despite aggressive intravenous crystalloid hydration and massive transfusion. Additional bridging intervention was needed to hold out blood pressure during transferring patient to angiography room. REBOA is an endovascular technique that can temporarily control bleeding from the branches of descending aorta. It can be a useful tool in critical situations like this case.

7.3 A Cardiogenic Shock Case due to ST-Elevation Myocardial Infarction

A 63-year-old male patient came to the emergency department (ED) with chest pain and dyspnea started 3 h ago. He had underlying diabetes mellitus. His initial vital signs were 82/34 mmHg–99 bpm–22 cpm–36.3 °C (saturation at 81%). Physical examination revealed jugular vein engorgement and crackle in both basal lung fields. His initial ECG was as above (Fig. 7.9):

Q. What do you see in the initial ECG? Which type of MI do you suspect?

A. (1) Regular heart rate without evidence of arrhythmia; (2) ST elevation in lead III and V1–5 and reciprocal changes in lead I, aVL, and V6, which is suggestive of STEMI involving anterior wall.

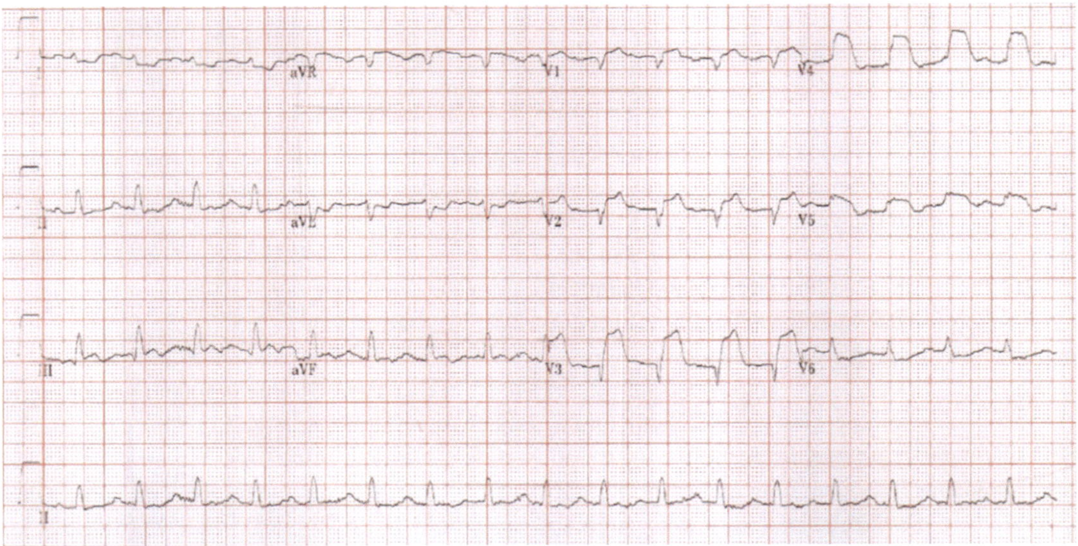

Fig. 7.9 Initial electrocardiography of the patient

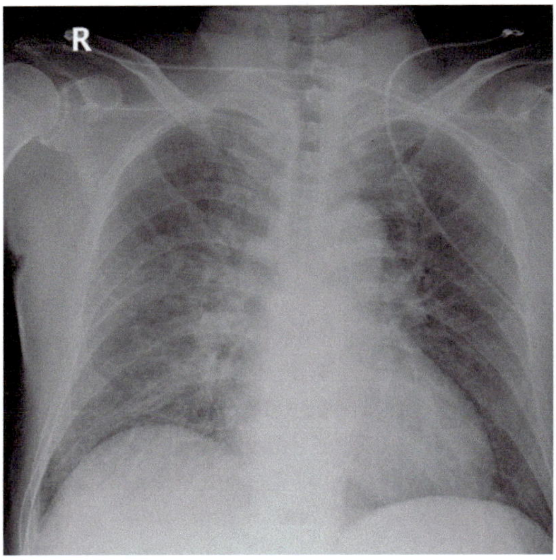

Fig. 7.10 Initial chest X-ray of the patient

Continuous monitoring of blood pressure, heart rate, and SpO2 was started. Rapid crystalloid infusion with 500 mL of normal saline and oxygen administration were also started. Cardiologist was called in and the patient was given aspirin, clopidogrel, and cholesterol-lowering statin drug. During fluid resuscitation, chest X-ray was taken (Fig. 7.10).

Q. What do you see in the initial chest X-ray? Please discuss about the clinical significance of the finding.

A. Chest X-ray showed pulmonary congestion. Fluid resuscitation should be avoided if there is pulmonary congestion. In this case, patient complained dyspnea and SpO_2 was low. In addition, chest X-ray showed pulmonary edema. Thus, administration of fluid should be cautious not to compromise respiration.

Bedside echocardiography revealed low ejection fraction (estimated as less than 30%) and hypokinesia in mid-anteroseptal and whole apical wall. Meanwhile his initial laboratory results came out.

Arterial blood gas analysis			CBC			Chemistry			Cardiac enzyme			Coagulation panel			Urinalysis		
pH	7.366		WBC	19,820	/μL	Na	134	mmol/L	CK		ng/mL	PT (%)	89	%	WBC	1–4	/HPF
pCO2	42.6	mmHg	Hb	15.9	g/dL	K	4.1	mmol/L	CK-MB	7.1	ng/mL	PT (INR)	1.09	INR	RBC	1–4	/HPF
pO2	56.1	mmHg	Hct	48.6	%	Cl	100	mmol/L	TnI	0.283	pg/mL	aPTT	31.4	Seconds	Albumin	Negative	
HCO3-	22.8	mmol/L	Platelet	232,000	/μL	TCO2	22	mmol/L	BNP	163.5	pg/dL	D-dimer	0.76	μg/mL	Nitrite	Negative	
Base excess	NA	mmol/L				BUN	23	mg/dL				Fibrinogen	463	mg/dL	Bacteria	Negative	
Lactate	2.4	mmol/L				Cr	1.21	mg/dL									
						AST	150	IU/L									
						ALT	127	IU/L									
						T.bil	1.4	mg/dL									
						ALP	385	IU/L									
						T.prot.	5.8	g/dL									
						Albumin	3.5	g/dL									

After initial administration of isotonic crystalloid (500 mL), blood pressure was 85/44 mmHg.

Q. What is your resuscitation plan for hypotension?

A. Since the contractility of left ventricle was decreased and return of blood from lungs was impaired, fluid administration would cause more congestions. The amount of blood returning to the heart should be reduced and vasopressors are preferred to fluid resuscitation.

Vasopressors like dopamine, norepinephrine, and epinephrine can be used to maintain adequate blood pressure. The target mean blood pressure for adequate splanchnic and renal perfusion is based on clinical indices of organ function (MAP $\geq$ 65 mmHg). Dopamine increases myocardial contractility and constricts blood vessel, but increases myocardial oxygen demand. Dobutamine does not increase myocardial oxygen demand, but can increase heart rate and peripheral vasodilation. Thus, dobutamine can be used to increase cardiac output if blood pressure is maintained.

Intravenous infusion of dopamine was started at a rate of 5 μg/kg/min and was titrated up to 20 μg/kg/min to maintain mean blood pressure over 65 mmHg. He was transferred to cath lab and CAG and primary PCI were performed. Coronary angiography showed total occlusion in proximal left anterior descending (LAD) artery and diffuse stenosis at distal LAD and proximal left circumflex (LCX) artery. Thrombosuction and ballooning was followed by stenting which was performed into LAD (Fig. 7.11).

His diagnosis was made as acute myocardial infarction caused by two coronary diseases (LAD and LCX).

During coronary catheterization, blood pressure dropped gradually and norepinephrine infusion was started. Immediately after coronary catheterization, saturation decreased to 81% despite oxygen supply with a rate of 12 L/min. Repeated chest radiography showed aggravation of pulmonary edema (Fig. 7.12).

High-flow nasal cannula was applied at a flow of 50 L/min with FiO_2 of 60%, but blood pressure decreased to 82/32 mmHg and the patient complained shortness of breath. His SpO_2 was dropped to less than 80% despite increased FiO_2 up to 80% (Fig. 7.13).

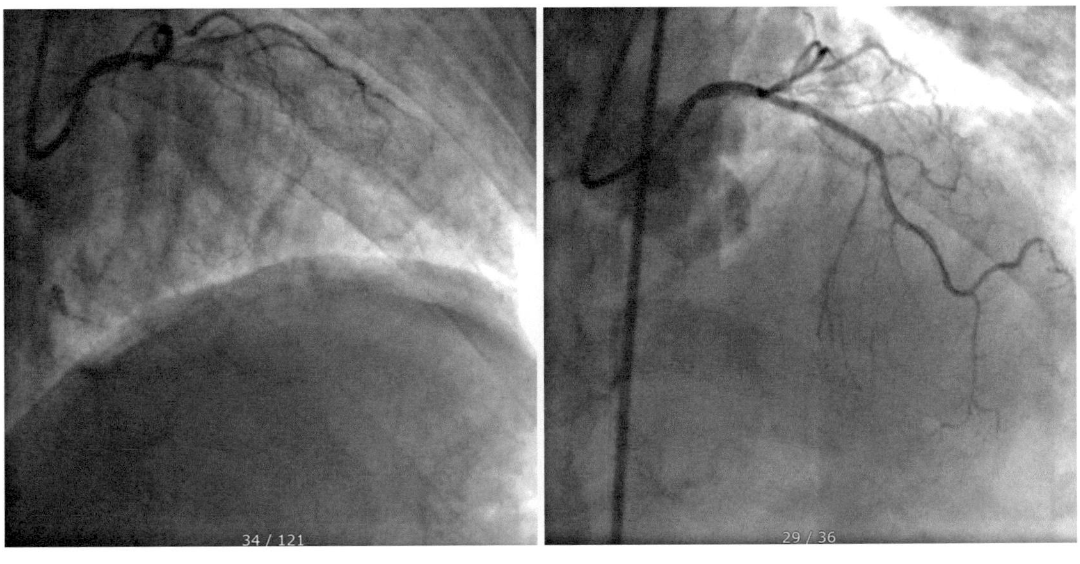

Fig. 7.11 Total thrombotic occlusion of LAD (left). Reperfusion after PCI (right)

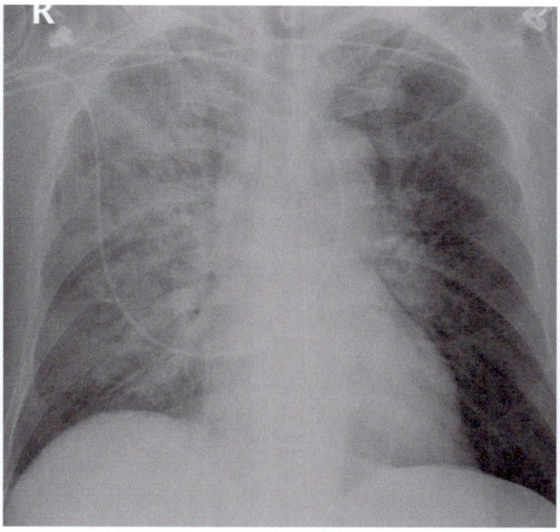

Fig. 7.12 A repeated chest X-ray of the patient showing significant pulmonary edema

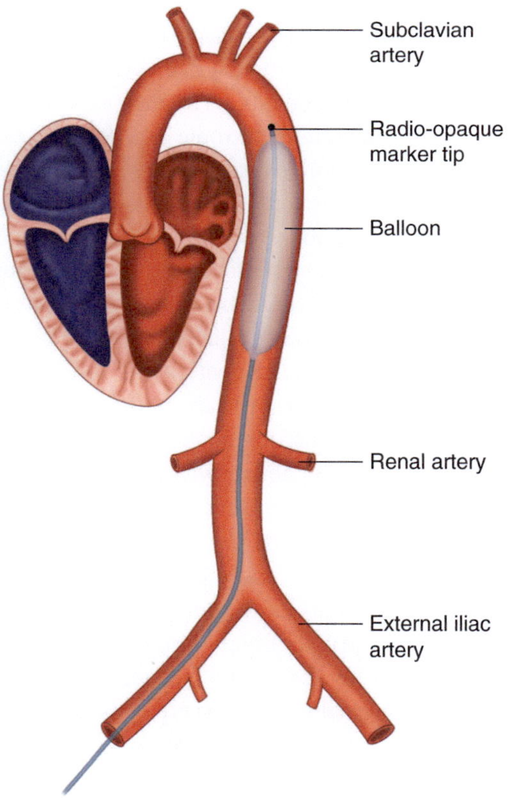

Fig. 7.13 Intra-aortic balloon pump (IABP) placement. The usual route is common femoral artery. The radio-opaque distal end is positioned in the proximal descending aorta

Q. What is your strategy for refractory shock and desaturation in LV failure?

A. Advanced airway placement and application of mechanical ventilation should be considered in the case of desaturation and patient deterioration. Intra-aortic balloon pump (IABP) may be considered as a temporizing measure in complicated myocardial infarction. This device can increase cardiac output, reduce afterload cardiac contractility and oxygen demand, and improve coronary artery blood flow.

He was admitted to coronary intensive care unit (ICU) for hemodynamic monitoring and application of ventilator. After 5 h of reperfusion therapy, ST segment and T wave of ECG were normalized (Fig. 7.14).

After stabilization of blood pressure, furosemide was administrated intravenously to control pulmonary edema. After 24 h of the reperfusion therapy, chest radiography showed decreased pulmonary edema. IABP was weaned off (Fig. 7.15).

He was treated with furosemide till improvement of pulmonary edema. He gradually improved over several days of hospital stay and discharged with prescriptions of dual-antiplatelet agents, beta-blocker, and cholesterol-lowering statin.

7.3.1 Summary

This case represents cardiogenic shock caused by left ventricular failure. Initial resuscitation of cardiogenic shock includes adequate oxygenation, fluid administration to correct hypovolemia, and hemodynamic optimization using vasopressors or inotropes. Adequate oxygenation to prevent further myocardial and systemic ischemia is

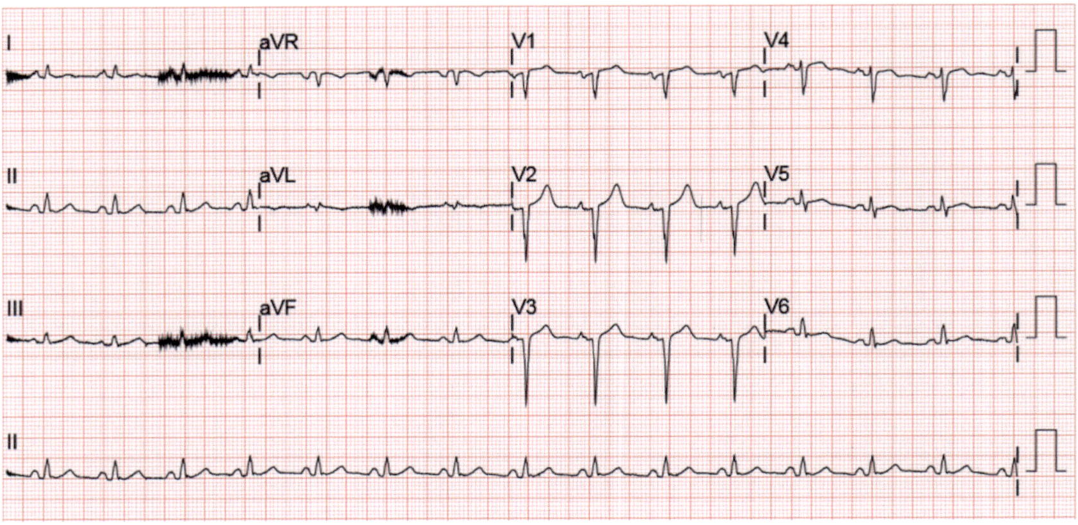

Fig. 7.14 Normalized ST elevation after reperfusion therapy

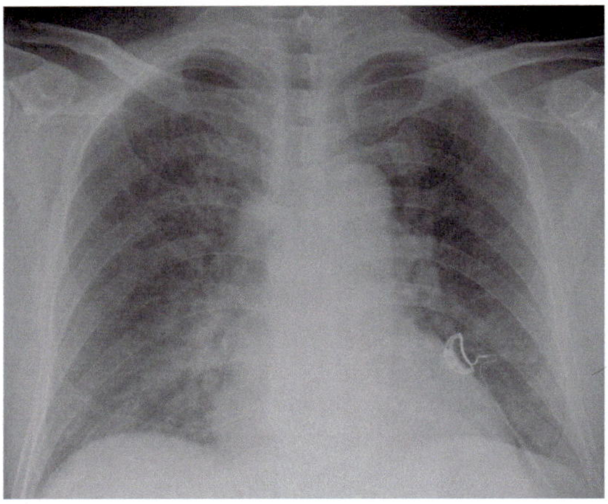

Fig. 7.15 Decreased pulmonary edema after diuresis

important. Usually, patients with cardiogenic shock caused by LV failure present with pulmonary edema and it can complicate adequate oxygenation. Thus, continuous monitoring of pulse oximetry is required. Intubation and mechanical ventilation are often required in severe cases. Positive pressure ventilation can improve pulmonary edema, but compromise venous return resulting in diminished LV preload.

In most patients with cardiogenic shock, fluid resuscitation is required. However, it can compromise respiration and care must be taken not to administer fluid excessively. Vasopressors or inotropes are used to preserve organ perfusion. The target mean blood pressure to maintain adequate splanchnic and renal perfusion is mean arterial pressure ≥65 mmHg, which is based on clinical indices of organ function. Patients with organ hypoperfusion require inotropic and/or vasopressor therapy. Dopamine increases myocardial contractility and constricts blood vessels. On the other hand, dopamine may increase myocardial oxygen requirement, which results in further myocardial ischemia. Dobutamine also increases myocardial contractility, dilates peripheral blood vessels, and augments peripheral perfusion. However, it can increase heart rate and result in myocardial oxygen requirement.

In this case, dopamine was used to elevate and maintain blood pressure but failed to maintain blood pressure and oxygen saturation was dropped. Additional vasopressors like norepinephrine or addition of dobutamine can be used. Intra-aortic balloon pump (IABP) can also be used because IABP reduces LV afterload and augments coronary perfusion pressure, which can increase cardiac output and coronary blood flow. IABP is a useful adjunctive treatment to stabilize patients with cardiogenic shock. It is not a definitive treatment of myocardial infarction, but just a bridging therapy. Definitive diagnostic and therapeutic interventions should be performed after stabilization of patients using IABP.

7.4 A Cardiogenic Shock Case Due to RV Infarction

An 83-year-old female visited the emergency department (ED) complaining of ongoing chest discomfort which began 1 h before. The pain was somewhat severe (7 in NRS scale) and located at lower substernal area without radiation. Her initial vital signs were 95/37 mmHg–62 bpm–18 cpm–37.3 °C and oxygen saturation was 96%. Physical examination revealed mild tenderness on palpation of right upper quadrant in the abdomen. Because of her chest pain, she was given a tablet of nitroglycerin sublingually by the triage nurse. After 2 min, she became drowsy with BP of 56/33 mmHg.

Her 12-lead ECG taken during the triage was reviewed retrospectively by the ED staff and is presented below (Fig. 7.16).

Right precordial lead ECG was taken thereafter. There were ST elevations in lead V3R-6R which is suggestive of right ventricular involvement (Fig. 7.17).

Q. What are the abnormal findings of this ECG?

A. ST elevation in lead II, III, and aVF and reciprocal changes in lead I and aVL. ST depression in precordial lead (lead V2–6) → indicates inferior wall STEMI; irregular heart rate indicates atrial fibrillation; and subtle ST elevation in lead V1 and STE in lead III > II may suggest RV infarction.

Q. Was the use of nitroglycerin appropriate?

A. Giving nitroglycerin to those with possible RV infarction (including those with ST changes in the inferior leads) should be avoided because RV infarction causes decreased preload. Nitroglycerin can further decrease the preload and can cause profound shock.

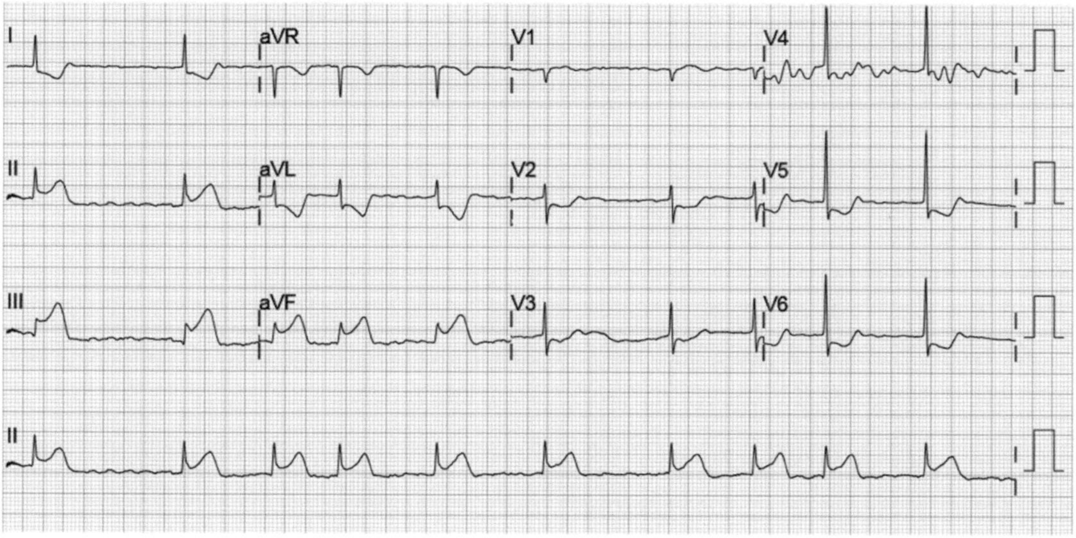

Fig. 7.16 Initial ECG of the patient, ST elevation in the inferior leads, and reciprocal changes in the anterolateral leads

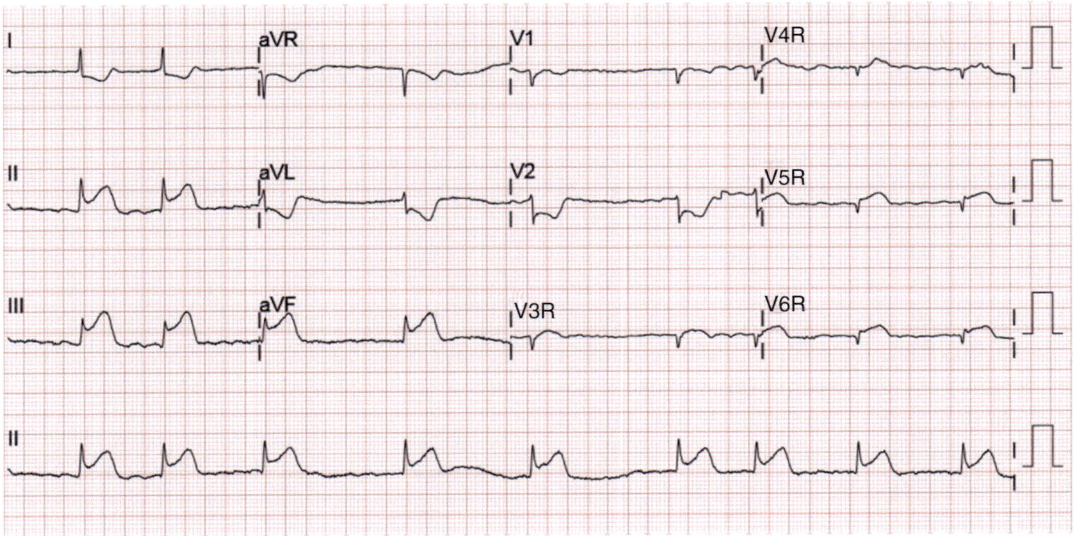

Fig. 7.17 Reverse electrocardiography of the patient. V3R-6R ST elevation suggests RV infarction

Q. Please describe how to interpret "reverse" ECG.

A. The reverse ECG is obtained by placing the precordial lead on the right anterior chest as shown in the following figure.

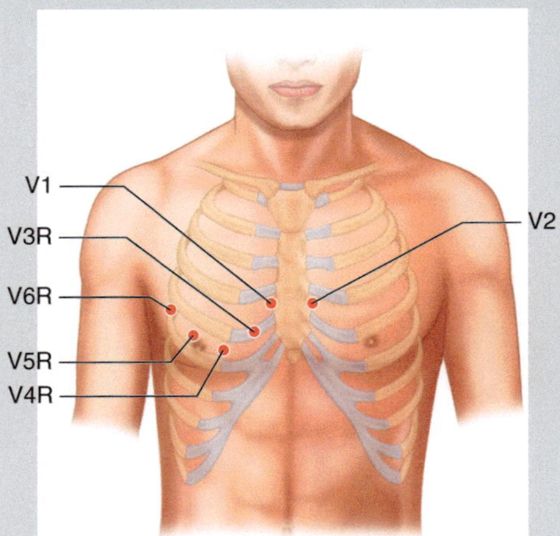

These right-sided precordial leads provide electrical information about the right side of the heart that is difficult to obtain from conventional ECG. The most useful lead is V4R, which is obtained by placing the V4 electrode in the fifth right intercostal space in the midclavicular line. ST elevation in V4R has a sensitivity of 88%, specificity of 78%, and diagnostic accuracy of 83% in the diagnosis of RV MI.

Meanwhile, her initial laboratory results were reported. The troponin I level was in normal range and initial chest X-ray showed no significant lung lesion.

Arterial blood gas analysis			CBC			Chemistry			Cardiac enzyme			Coagulation panel			Urinalysis		
pH	7.38		WBC	10,700	/μL	Na	138	mmol/L	CK	35	ng/mL	PT (INR)	1.14	INR	WBC	NA	/HPF
pCO2	28	mmHg	Hb	10.8	g/dL	K	4.4	mmol/L	CK-MB	<1.0	ng/mL	aPTT	35.5	Seconds	RBC	NA	/HPF
pO2	59	mmHg	Hct	31.3	%	Cl	102	mmol/L	TnI	<0.035	pg/mL	D-dimer	3.47	μg/mL	Albumin	NA	
HCO3-	19	mmol/L	Platelet	251,000	/μL	TCO2	22	mmol/L	Pro-BNP	430.7	pg/dL				Nitrite	NA	
Base excess	NA	mmol/L				BUN	20	mg/dL							Bacteria	NA	
Lactate	NA	mmol/L				Cr	1.01	mg/dL									
						AST	160	IU/L									
						ALT	56	IU/L									
						T.bil	0.7	mg/dL									
						ALP	112	IU/L									
						T.prot.	NA	g/dL									
						Albumin	3.4	g/dL									

Initially she was in shock (defined by SBP <90 mmHg); thus, resuscitation with isotonic crystalloid and primary PCI was planned. After administration of isotonic crystalloid (1500 mL), she was still in shock (BP 82/43 mmHg) and bedside echocardiography revealed dilated RV and normal systolic function of LV. Interventricular septum was deviated to the left side.

Q. What is your fluid resuscitation plan at this time?

A. RV failure limits Lt heart filling through the mechanism of decreased RV CO. Thus, fluid administration is critical to adequate RV filling to maintain adequate LV filling. However, vigorous fluid administration can result in very high RV end-diastolic pressure, and thus can shift interventricular septum to LV cavity, which can result in impairment of LV filling. Thus, fluid administration should be careful and frequent assessment of CO with fluid administration is required.

Administration of fluid was stopped and then dobutamine was administered at a dose of 10 μg/kg/min. Her blood pressure was elevated to 95/50 mmHg and heart rate was increased to 95 bpm.

Q. If the patient's blood pressure is not adequately elevated after administration of fluid and inotropes, what will you do next?

A. If hypotension was persisted even after administration of adequate amount of fluid and inotropes, one should consider the possibilities of mechanical complications such as ventricular wall rupture. A quick bedside echocardiography may be useful to rule out it.

The patient was prepared for primary PCI (including administration of dual-antiplatelet agents), and then was transferred to cath lab. Coronary angiography revealed total occlusion of right coronary artery (left). Primary PCI was performed (right) (Figs. 7.18 and 7.19).

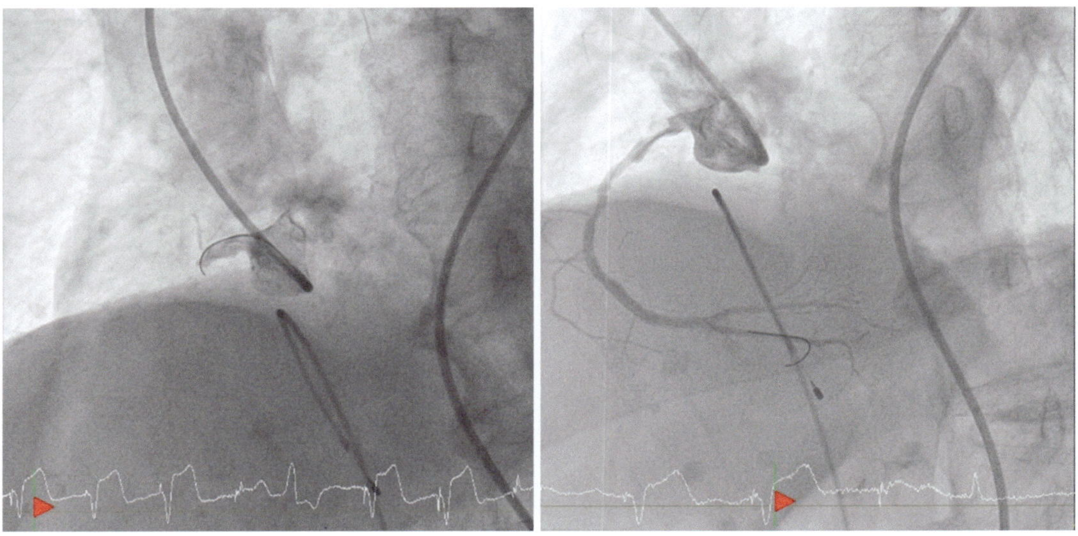

Fig. 7.18 Occluded right coronary artery (left) reperfused after PCI (right)

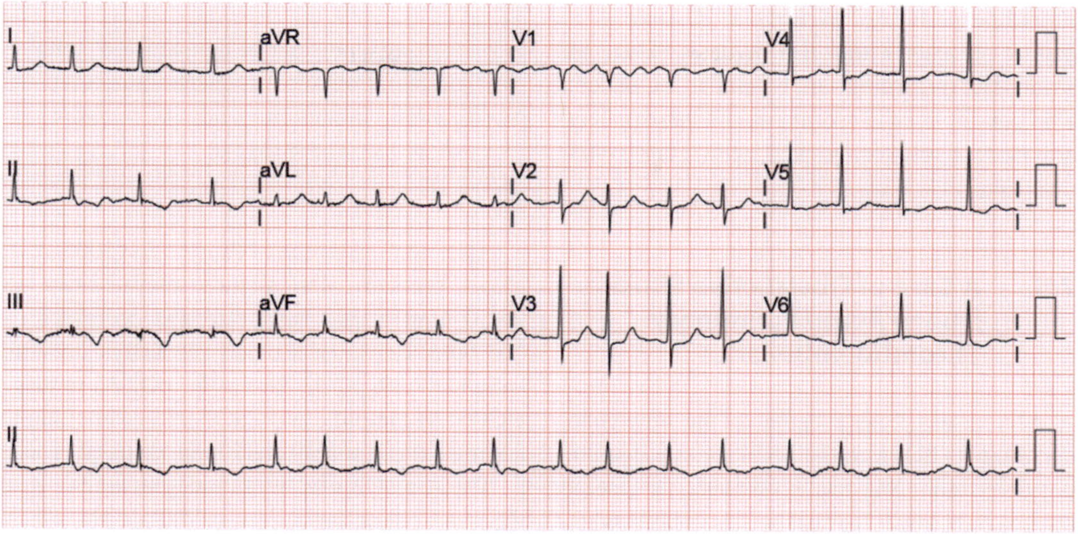

Fig. 7.19 The ECG taken after PCI, the ST elevations were resolved

After PCI, her blood pressure increased to 110/80 mmHg and the dobutamine infusion was tapered off. Her ECG showed complete resolution of ST elevation. The patient was treated for 3 days in ICU and then was discharged after additional 2 days of stays in general ward.

7.4.1 Summary

This is a case of cardiogenic shock resulted from RV infarction. Acute myocardial infarction is the most important cause of cardiogenic shock. RV infarction usually has different pathophysiology of shock. Failure of RV stroke work results in diminished LV filling, and thus diminished LV preload. Thus, initial resuscitation of shock caused by RV failure requires relatively large amount of fluid to increase and maintain LV preload, which is different with cardiogenic shock caused by LV failure. Usually vigorous fluid resuscitation in LV failure increases LV workload and aggravates myocardial ischemia and pulmonary edema. However, excessive fluid administration in RV infarction results in increased RV end-diastolic pressure, which can deviate interventricular septum to left ventricle and results in impairment of LV filling. Thus, frequent assessment of cardiac output during initial fluid resuscitation should be performed. If cardiac output and blood pressure are not maintained after administration of adequate amount of fluid (adequate RV end-diastolic pressure), inotropic therapy can be considered. Dobutamine, milrinone, levosimendan, norepinephrine, and low-dose vasopressin can be used. When the patient is still hemodynamically unstable after administration of adequate fluid and inotropics, mechanical complication of RV infarction (ventricular wall rupture, cardiac tamponade, etc.) should be considered. Bedside echocardiography is a useful tool to assess mechanical complication of myocardial infarction. For definite treatment of RV infarction, percutaneous coronary intervention should be performed as early as possible if the patient presents within 6 h of onset. There are scant data regarding improvement in patients who present after 12 h of onset and these patients are more likely being well with conservative management.

7.5 A Case of Obstructive Shock Due to Acute Pulmonary Thromboembolism

A 42-year-old female came to the emergency department (ED) through EMS for syncope during defecation. She had no underlying disease, but her right lower leg had been immobilized for 5 days due to ankle sprain. At the time of ED arrival, blood pressure was 75/40 mmHg, heart rate was 127 bpm, respiratory rate was 28 cpm, and body temperature was 35.7 °C. The pulse oximetry revealed SpO2 of 92% while maintaining oxygen supply at 6 L/min via nasal prong. She was alert, but complained of dizziness and dyspnea.

Physical examination revealed no abnormal breathing sound, but slightly engorged jugular vein and right-leg swelling. Continuous monitoring of blood pressure, heart rate, and SpO2 was started, fluid bolus was administered, and oxygen was administered via nasal prong at a rate of 6 L/min.

Q. What is your different diagnoses?

A. The patient was afebrile and there was no abnormal breathing sound. However, she had dyspnea, profound hypotension, and tachycardia. Considering her recent immobilization of right lower leg, pulmonary embolism should be the first differential diagnosis. Other conditions causing profound hypotension and desaturation such as pneumonia, myocardial infarction, and heart failure should also be ruled out.

After administration of fluid bolus (1000 mL), blood pressure was slightly elevated up to 85/50 mmHg, and heart rate was decreased to 105 bpm. Her arterial blood gas analysis results were pH 7.39, pCO2 32 mmHg, pO2 65 mmHg, HCO3 20 mmol/L, and SaO2 92% while maintaining oxygen supply at 6 L/min via nasal prong.

The A-aDO2 was 59.0 mmHg assuming that the atmospheric pressure was 760 mmHg which indicates increased A-a DO2 that usually results from ventilation-perfusion mismatch or right-to-left shunt.

Q. What is A-aDO2? Please describe how to calculate it and interpret the results.

A. The alveolar–arterial gradient (A-aO2, or A–a gradient) is a measure of the difference between the alveolar concentration (A) of oxygen and the arterial (a) concentration of oxygen. It is used in diagnosing the source of hypoxemia.

PA-aO2 = PAO2 - PaO2 (normal range: 10–25 mm Hg in room air, 30–50 mm Hg with 100% O2).

Elevated value of A-aDO2 means that oxygen is not effectively transferred from the alveoli to the blood. This includes V/Q mismatches such as PTE or R-L shunt.

Her first ECG was taken. The ECG showed sinus tachycardia and S wave in lead I, Q wave in lead III, and T wave inversion in lead III (S1Q3T3) (Fig. 7.20).

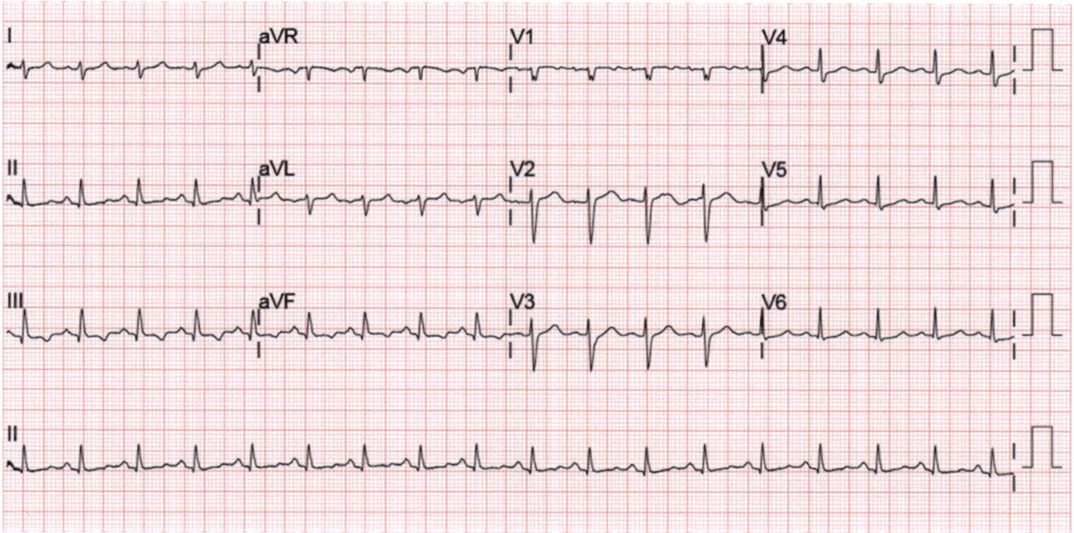

Fig. 7.20 Initial ECG of the patient, RV strain pattern (S1Q3T3) was observed

Q. What does the result of the ECG indicate?

A. The most common ECG finding in the setting of a pulmonary embolism is sinus tachycardia. However, the "S1Q3T3" pattern can be observed in patients with significant RV strain. The sign consists of a large S wave in lead I, a Q wave in lead III, and an inverted T wave in lead III. This pattern only occurs in about 10% of people with pulmonary embolisms.

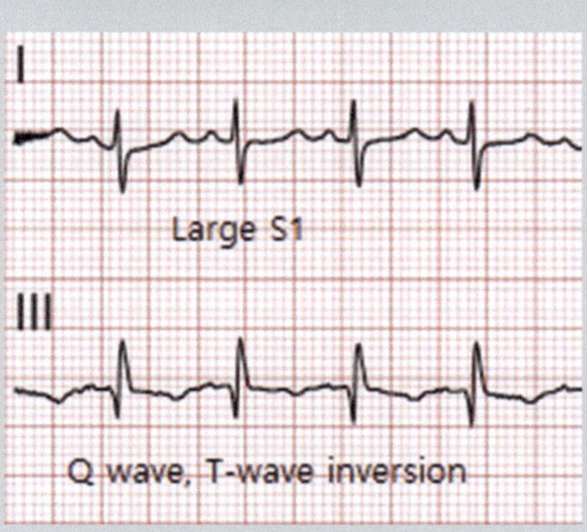

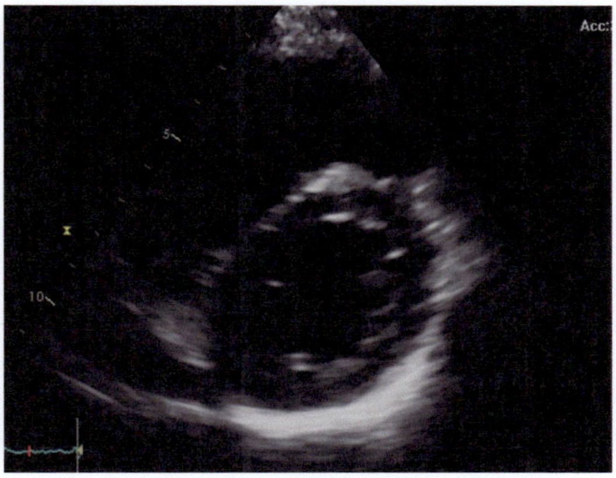

Fig. 7.21 The large RV cross-sectional area and the flattened interventricular septum ("D-shape" of LV) indicate RV strain

Bedside echocardiography was performed during initial resuscitation. It revealed dilated RV and severe TR, and D-shape LV (Fig. 7.21).

Meanwhile her initial laboratory results came out.

Arterial blood gas analysis			CBC			Chemistry			Cardiac enzyme			Coagulation panel			Urinalysis		
pH	7.390		WBC	16,910	/μL	Na	140	mmol/L	CK		ng/mL	PT (%)	84	%	WBC	NA	/HPF
pCO2	32	mmHg	Hb	14.7	g/dL	K	4.5	mmol/L	CK-MB	2.1	ng/mL	PT (INR)	1.11	INR	RBC	NA	/HPF
pO2	65	mmHg	Hct	43.6	%	Cl	104	mmol/L	TnI	0.772	pg/mL	aPTT	37.1	Seconds	Albumin	NA	
HCO3-	20	mmol/L	Platelet	153,000	/μL	TCO2	21	mmol/L				D-dimer	>20	μg/mL	Nitrite	NA	
Base excess	NA	mmol/L				BUN	13	mg/dL				Fibrinogen	299	mg/dL	Bacteria	NA	
Lactate	NA	mmol/L				Cr	1.01	mg/dL									
						AST	405	IU/L									
						ALT	306	IU/L									
						T.bil	0.7	mg/dL									
						ALP	109	IU/L									
						T.prot.	8.0	g/dL									
						Albumin	4.0	g/dL									

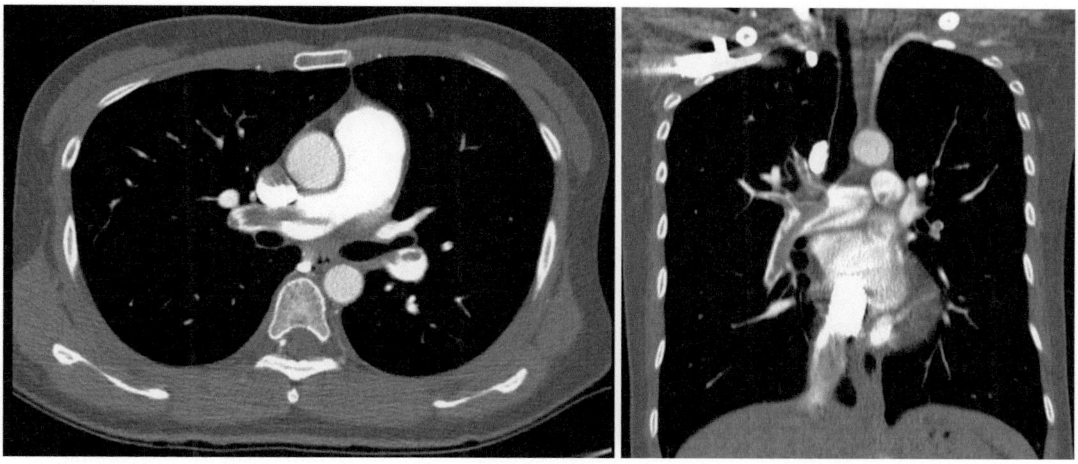

Fig. 7.22 Thrombotic occlusion of right main pulmonary trunk

It confirms RV strain and is suggestive of RV outflow obstruction. Therefore, massive pulmonary embolism was suspected. To confirm the presumptive diagnosis, contrast-enhanced chest CT scan was done while continuing fluid resuscitation and shown below (Fig. 7.22).

Q. What is your management plan considering the pulmonary thromboembolism, RV strain, and obvious shock?

A. Acute thrombolysis using IV thrombolytics should be considered because of her obvious hemodynamic instability.

Thrombolysis Therapy for Acute Pulmonary Embolism

1. Indications
   - The only widely accepted indication for systemic thrombolysis: Persistent hypotension or shock (i.e., a systolic blood pressure <90 mmHg or a decrease in the systolic blood pressure by ≥40 mmHg from baseline)
2. Potential indications for thrombolytic therapy in venous thromboembolism
   - High-risk (massive) PE, i.e., presence of hypotension related to PE*
   - Presence of severe hypoxemia (particularly in those with a contribution from concomitant cardiopulmonary disease)
   - Patients with acute PE who appear to be decompensating but are not yet hypotensive
   - Patients with severe right ventricular dysfunction and tachycardia due to PE
   - Clot in transit (i.e., right atrium or ventricle)
   - Extensive deep vein thrombosis
3. Absolute contraindications
   - Prior intracranial hemorrhage
   - Known structural cerebral vascular lesion
   - Known malignant intracranial neoplasm
   - Ischemic stroke within 3 months (excluding stroke within 3 h*)
   - Suspected aortic dissection
   - Active bleeding or bleeding diathesis (excluding menses)
   - Significant closed-head trauma or facial trauma within 3 months
4. Relative contraindications
   - History of chronic, severe, poorly controlled hypertension
   - Severe uncontrolled hypertension on presentation (SBP > 180 mmHg or DBP > 110 mmHg)
   - History of ischemic stroke more than 3 months prior

- Traumatic or prolonged (>10 min) CPR or major surgery less than 3 weeks
- Recent (within 2–4 weeks) internal bleeding
- Noncompressible vascular punctures
- Recent invasive procedure
- For streptokinase/anistreplase: Prior exposure (more than 5 days ago) or prior allergic reaction to these agents
- Pregnancy
- Active peptic ulcer
- Pericarditis or pericardial fluid
- Current use of anticoagulant (e.g., warfarin sodium) that has produced an elevated international normalized ratio (INR) >1.7 or prothrombin time (PT) >15 s
- Age > 75 years
- Diabetic retinopathy

5. Regimen
   - Alteplase: 10 mg bolus infusion → followed by 90 mg (+NS500 mL) over 2 h

After confirming the diagnosis of pulmonary thromboembolism, 10 mg of rtPA was infused over 10 min, followed by 90 mg over 2 h. After thrombolysis infusion, she was admitted to ICU for 1 day. Her vital signs were stabilized gradually and then transferred to general ward (Fig. 7.23).

She was discharged with a prescription of rivaroxaban (NOAC) to maintain anticoagulation.

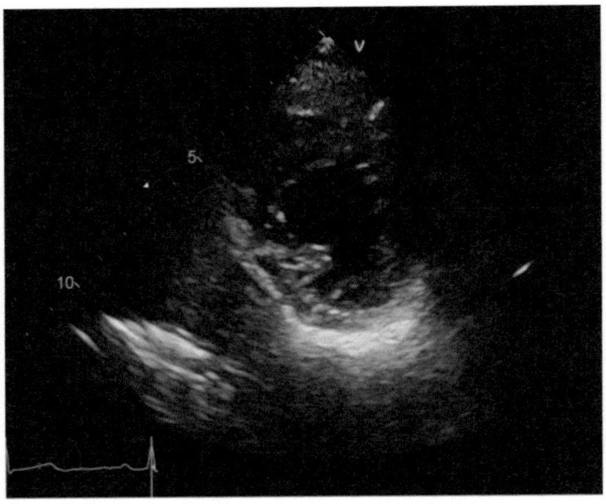

Fig. 7.23 The axial view of left ventricle at hospital day 7, the D-shape appearance has disappeared

7.5.1 Summary

This case is an example of obstructive shock. Pulmonary thromboembolism causes RV outflow tract obstruction, resulting in diminished LV filling. As a consequence, cardiac output decreases and hypotension occurs. As a result of decreased preload, tachycardia can be occurred as a compensatory mechanism. In addition, increased cardiac workload in right ventricle results in RV strain, which can result in ECG change of RV strain (typically S1Q3T3 pattern). Initial resuscitation includes correction of hypovolemia and respiratory support. Although angiographic CT scan of chest can make a confirmative diagnosis of PTE, it is sometimes hard to perform due to hemodynamic instability. Bedside echocardiography is a useful tool to identify the cause of shock and it can detect the findings of RV strain, deviation of interventricular septum (D-shape LV), and sometimes thrombus in pulmonary trunk. The treatment of PTE includes anticoagulation for preventing further formation of thrombus and resolution of thrombus by thrombolytics or mechanical thrombectomy. Usually, mechanical thrombectomy is hard to perform in hemodynamically unstable patients, because it requires transport of patients to operation room or angiography room. In addition, there are many case reports that ECMO can be a temporizing measure in refractory cardiac arrest due to pulmonary embolism.

7.6 A Case of Obstructive Shock Due to Cardiac Tamponade

An 81-year-old female with a history of hypertension and dyslipidemia came to the emergency department (ED) for chest pain. Before the ED visit, she had visited oriental medicine clinic because of headache and epigastric discomfort. Her chest pain began after the practitioner at the clinic performed an acupuncture to her chest. She fainted after the onset of chest pain and was promptly brought to the ED by EMS vehicle. On physical examination, there was a long acupuncture needle deeply inserted at the fourth left intercostal space of sternal border (the photo could not be taken because the clerk from the oriental medicine clinic removed it without permission from ED staffs). She was confused and diaphoretic. Her initial vital signs were 71/52 mmHg–106 bpm–24 cpm–36.3 °C. Lung sounds were clear and symmetric. Heart sound was a little muffled without a murmur or gallop. There was no abdominal tenderness.

Q. What will you do for initial resuscitation?

A. Rapid accumulation of fluid in the pericardial space, which increases pressure of pericardial space and impairs relaxation and filling of the ventricles, resulting in reduced ventricular filling and hemodynamic compromise. Higher filling pressure and large amount of venous return will overcome increase in intrapericardial pressure.
Therefore, volume infusion using crystalloid or blood products to provide higher filling pressure would be the most important step.

Q. What is the most likely diagnosis?

A. She had hypotension, confusion, and diaphoresis which indicate hemodynamic unstability. Because her symptoms developed after chest trauma (deep needle insertion), both cardiac tamponade and tension pneumothorax should be considered as possible diagnoses. The patient had muffled heart sound without decrease in lung sound; the most likely diagnosis would be acute cardiac tamponade.

After initial fluid administration, her blood pressure was increased a little, but after a while became low again as 67/42 mmHg. Meanwhile, her initial laboratory reports came out.

Arterial blood gas analysis			CBC			Chemistry			Cardiac enzyme			Coagulation panel			Urinalysis		
pH	7.502		WBC	9630	/μL	Na	138	mmol/L	CK		ng/mL	PT (%)	87.6	%	WBC	<1	/HPF
pCO2	23.4	mmHg	Hb	11.7	g/dL	K	3.6	mmol/L	CK-MB	0.7	ng/mL	PT (INR)	1.07	INR	RBC	<1	/HPF
pO2	109.7	mmHg	Hct	35.0	%	Cl	104.4	mmol/L	TnI	0.131	pg/mL	aPTT	30.0	Seconds	Albumin	Negative	
HCO3-	17.9	mmol/L	Platelet	290,000	/μL	TCO2	16.8	mmol/L				D-dimer	1.15	μg/mL	Nitrite	Negative	
Base excess	NA	mmol/L				BUN	18	mg/dL				Fibrinogen	NA	mg/dL	Bacteria	Negative	
Lactate	3.38	mmol/L				Cr	0.89	mg/dL									
						AST	35	IU/L									
						ALT	34	IU/L									
						T.bil	0.5	mg/dL									
						ALP	74	IU/L									
						T.prot.	6.1	g/dL									
						Albumin	3.6	g/dL									

There was no active lung lesion or cardiomegaly on her initial chest X-ray. There was also no significant abnormality except sinus tachycardia in her initial electrocardiogram. Her bedside echocardiography found moderate amount of pericardial effusion and diastolic RV collapse. The treating physician made a presumptive diagnosis of traumatic cardiac tamponade due to hemopericardium and a cardiac surgeon was consulted promptly (Figs. 7.24 and 7.25).

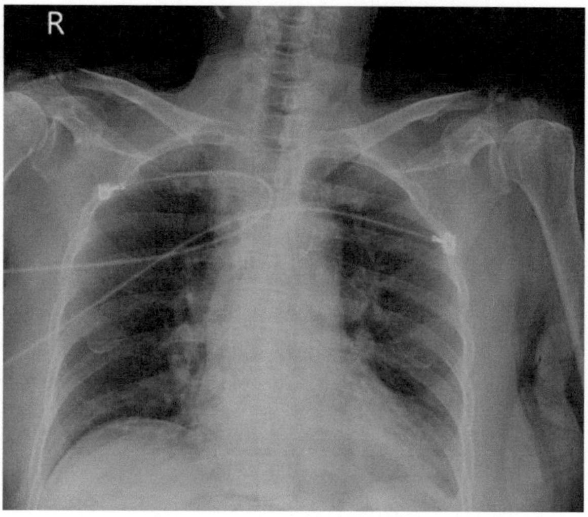

Fig. 7.24 Initial chest X-ray of the patient. Significant increase in heart size was not observed

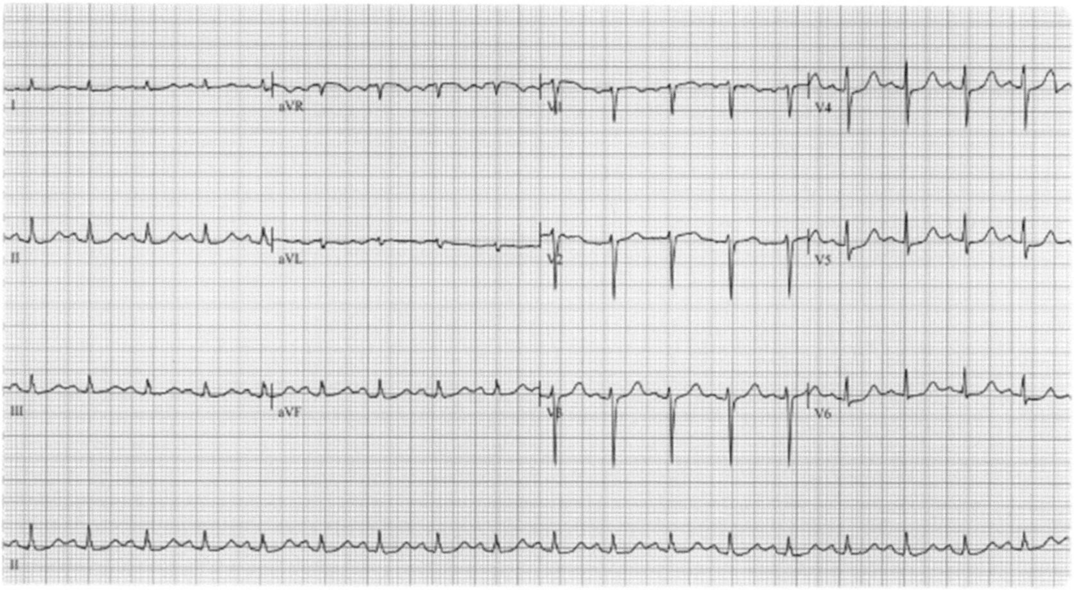

Fig. 7.25 Initial electrocardiogram of the patient which was nonspecific

Q. The chest image and electrocardiogram showed no signs of cardiac tamponade (e.g., enlarged cardiac silhouette, low voltage, or electrical alternans). Discuss about the diagnostic performances of chest PA and ECG in cardiac tamponade.

A. Both chest X-ray and electrocardiogram are not sensitive to cardiac tamponade. One of the reasons is the dependence of the development of cardiac tamponade on the rapidity of pericardial fluid accumulation. With chronic accumulation of a pericardial effusion, pericardial compliance increases gradually. However, rapid accumulation does not allow such increase in compliance and, in acute trauma like this case, small accumulation of blood in pericardial space can significantly increase intrapericardial pressure and be complicated by cardiac tamponade without significant abnormalities in chest X-ray.

Upper, enlarged cardiac silhouette; Lower, electrical alternans and low-voltage sign.

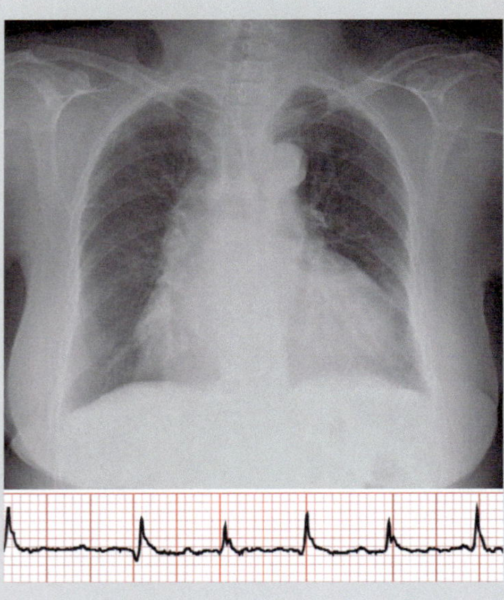

Q. What is diastolic RV collapse? Discuss about the echocardiographic findings of cardiac tamponade.

A. In cardiac tamponade, RV diastolic collapse can be observed during echocardiography in early diastole when the RV volume is still low. It is less sensitive but very specific compared to RA collapse.

After fluid resuscitation and monitoring with arterial line insertion, the patient was transferred to OR for emergency operation. In the operation room, the surgeons evacuated 300 cc of pericardial hematoma and repaired the small perforation at the right ventricle. The patient remained stable after the surgery and was discharged home without complication (Fig. 7.26).

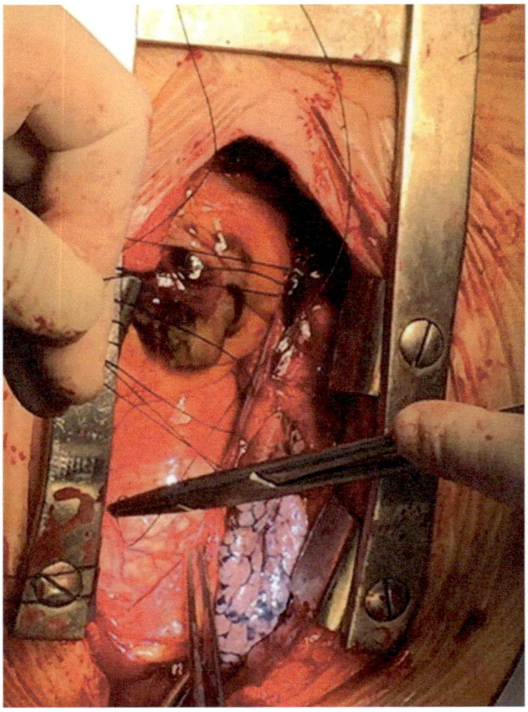

Fig. 7.26 After evacuation of 300 cc of pericardial hematoma, right ventricular perforation was identified and primary closure was done

7.6.1 Summary

Cardiac tamponade is one of the lethal causes of shock. The incidence of cardiac tamponade is two cases per 10,000 populations in the United States. The most common causes are malignant diseases and it accounts for 30–60% of the overall incidence. Although it is not a relatively common cause of shock, a physician should consider it as one of the many differential diagnoses of shock especially when malignancy, chronic kidney disease, and trauma are present. In this case, the cardiomegaly and characteristic ECG changes were not present. This could be due to the fast progression of pericardial filling by blood because the severity of the condition is also dependent on the speed of its development. This is commonly observed in traumatic cardiac tamponade. Approximately 2% of penetrating injuries are reported to result in cardiac tamponade. In this case, percutaneous drainage was not performed in the ED. It was because rapid operation by a thoracic surgeon was available. However, if prompt surgical intervention is impossible or delayed, emergency subxiphoid percutaneous drainage or echocardiographically guided pericardiocentesis must be performed.

7.7 A Septic Shock Case Due to Pneumonia

A 56-year-old woman visited the emergency department (ED) with chief complaint of vomiting. She had fever, chill, and yellowish sputum which began at the morning of her visit. She had underlying disease of hypertension and osteoporosis. Her initial vital signs were 69/47 mmHg–120 bpm–32 cpm–34.7 °C with sPO2 level of 92%. Two weeks ago, she had cough and whitish sputum which had spontaneously resolved. Her physical examination revealed decreased lung sound at left lower lung field.

Q. Describe your assessment of the patient based on the initial presentation.

A. The first symptoms the patient experienced were fever, chill, and productive cough which suggest respiratory infection. At the ED presentation, she had hypotension (SBP 69 mmHg) and tachypnea (32 bpm) and thus positive for two qSOFA components. Therefore, she was screened to be positive for sepsis. To determine whether this patient is in septic shock, we need to know the response to adequate fluid resuscitation and blood lactate measurement (see pages 59–61).

Q. What is your initial fluid resuscitation plan?

A. Patients with sepsis are often in relative hypovolemia. It is recommended to infuse at least 30 mL/kg of crystalloids within the first 3 h. It would be considerate to infuse the fluid in predefined size of bolus (e.g., 300–500 cc) while monitoring the response to the sequential boluses. For this patient, four 500 cc boluses of normal saline (65 × 30 = 1950 mL) were rapidly administered (see page 65).

During the fluid resuscitation, ceftriaxone and azithromycin were administered with a presumptive diagnosis of pneumonia after obtaining specimens for blood and respiratory cultures. After the initial fluid infusion, her blood pressure increased, but was still low as 72/54 mmHg. On bedside echocardiography, her IVC diameter of 2.0 cm and its respiratory collapse with forceful inspiration were less than 50% (Fig. 7.27).

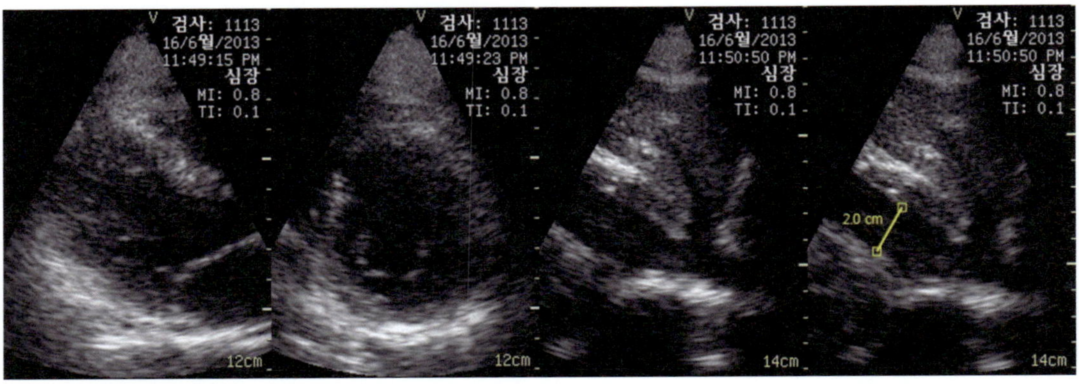

Fig. 7.27 Bedside ultrasonography findings

Q. Do we need further fluid resuscitation? If so, how will you do it?

A. Some patients with sepsis may require larger volume of fluid to achieve optimal hemodynamic status. Therefore, further fluid resuscitation should be considered. However, too much fluid can result in pulmonary edema. Therefore, fluid resuscitation for sepsis should be guided by hemodynamic assessment. SSC guideline recommends frequent reassessment of hemodynamic status using static or dynamic measurement.

- Static: CVP, PCWP, LV end-diastolic area by echocardiography, IVC diameter.
- Dynamic: Stroke volume variation, pulse pressure variation, passive leg raising (aortic blood flow, pulse pressure change, stroke volume change, cardiac output change), IVC collapsibility.

Bedside ultrasonography is a useful tool in monitoring volume status. The test identified "IVC plethora" in this patient. This suggests that adequate fluid resuscitation was achieved and there is a significant risk of pulmonary edema with further fluid administration. Because the patient is still hypotensive, initiation of vasopressors is required to achieve target mean arterial pressure of 65 mmHg.

Norepinephrine was started at the infusion rate of 8 μg/min. Meanwhile, her initial laboratory test results came out. The laboratory results indicate combined metabolic acidosis and respiratory alkalosis. The high CRP level indicates underlying inflammatory process.

Arterial blood gas analysis			CBC			Chemistry			Cardiac enzyme			Coagulation panel			Urinalysis		
pH	7.47		WBC	5200	/μL	Na	137	mmol/L	CK	NA	ng/mL	PT (Sec)	14.2	Seconds	WBC	<1	/HPF
pCO2	29	mmHg	Hb	10.7	g/dL	K	3.3	mmol/L	CK-MB	1.2	ng/mL	PT (INR)	1.31	INR	RBC	<1	/HPF
pO2	63	mmHg	Hct	32.3	%	Cl	102	mmol/L	TnI	0.01	pg/mL	aPTT	26.9	Seconds	Albumin	Trace	
HCO3-	23	mmol/L	Platelet	203,000	/μL	TCO2	23	mmol/L				D-dimer	1.63	μg/mL	Nitrite	Negative	
Base excess	NA	mmol/L				BUN	137	mg/dL				Fibrinogen	689	mg/dL	Bacteria	Negative	
Lactate	3.0	mmol/L				Cr	1.28	mg/dL									
						AST	94	IU/L									
						ALT	211	IU/L									
						T.bil	1.5	mg/dL									
						ALP	96	IU/L									
						T.prot.	5.6	g/dL									
						Albumin	2.9	g/dL									

Her electrocardiogram showed no significant arrhythmia or ST-T change. Her initial chest X-ray showed left lower lung field haziness (Fig. 7.28).

Her chest CT revealed airspace consolidation at her left lower lung field confirming the initial diagnosis of pneumonia (Fig. 7.29).

For infusion of vasopressors, central line was inserted through internal jugular vein. CVP was measured as 24 mmHg. ScvO2 was 59% and lactate level sampled in radial artery was 2.8 mmol/L. After starting norepinephrine at 8 μg/min, her blood pressure increased to 122/78 mmHg. However, her respiratory rate also increased to 33 cpm and the saturation was decreased to 85% with O2 flow rate of 6 L/min via facial mask. In follow-up echocardiography, decreased cardiac contractility was observed and IVC diameter was increased to 2.4 cm, with lesser proportion of collapse by respiration than before. Myocardial depression was suspected and dobutamine infusion was started at the rate of 5 μg/kg/min and O2 was increased to 10 L/min via facial mask (Fig. 7.30).

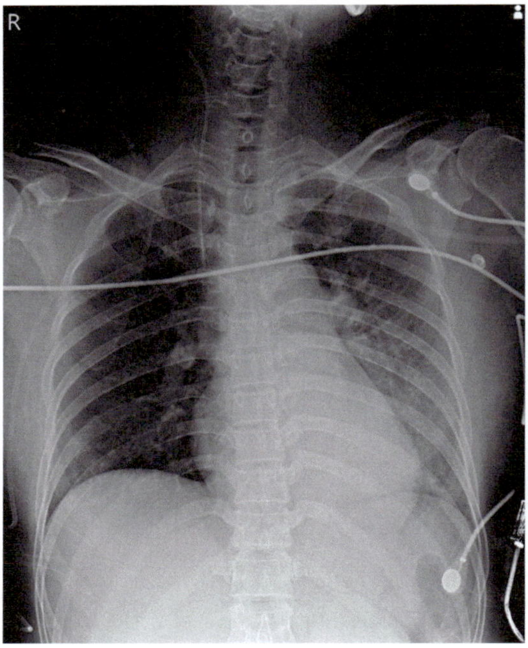

Fig. 7.28 There is haziness on left lower lung field

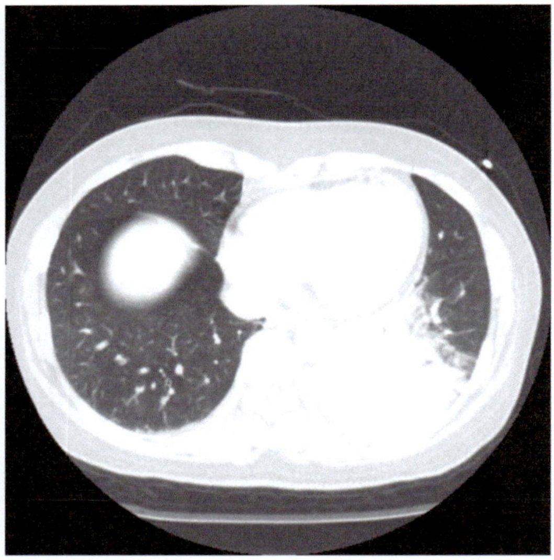

Fig. 7.29 There is dense consolidation located in the left lower lobe

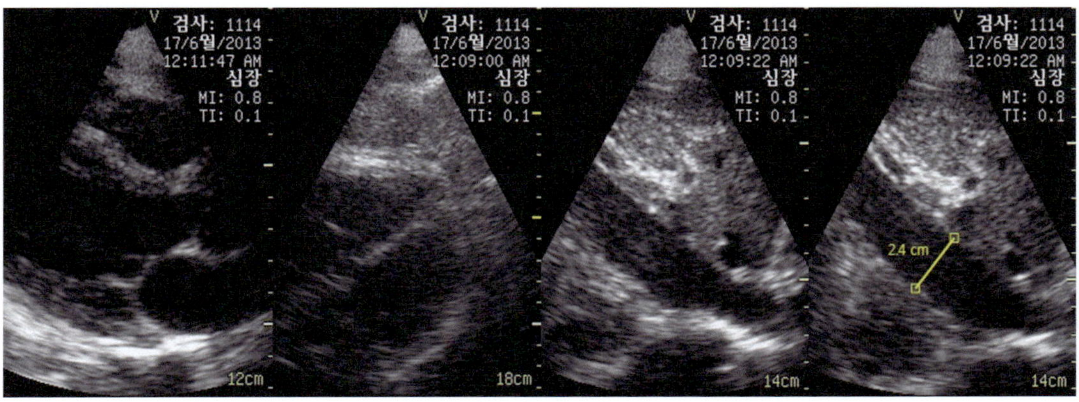

Fig. 7.30 Follow-up bedside (HD 2) ultrasonography showing increased IVC plethora and myocardial depression

Adrenergic Agents in Sepsis

Based on the SCC 2016 guideline, the first choice for the initial vasopressor should be norepinephrine in most cases. Dopamine can be used as an alternative agent in highly selected patient (low risk of tachyarrhythmia and absolute or relative bradycardia). Dobutamine can be used in case when there is persistent hypoperfusion.

(Surviving Sepsis Campaign: International Guidelines for Management of Sepsis and Septic Shock: 2016)

1. SSC guideline recommends norepinephrine as the first-choice vasopressor (strong recommendation, moderate quality of evidence).
2. SSC guideline suggests adding either vasopressin (up to 0.03 U/min) (weak recommendation, moderate quality of evidence) or epinephrine (weak recommendation, low quality of evidence) to norepinephrine with the intent of raising MAP to target, or adding vasopressin (up to 0.03 U/min) (weak recommendation, moderate quality of evidence) to decrease norepinephrine dosage.
3. SSC guideline suggests using dopamine as an alternative vasopressor agent to norepinephrine only in highly selected patients (e.g., patients with low risk of tachyarrhythmias and absolute or relative bradycardia) (weak recommendation, low quality of evidence).
4. SSC guideline recommends against using low-dose dopamine for renal protection (strong recommendation, high quality of evidence).
5. SSC guideline suggests using dobutamine in patients who show evidence of persistent hypoperfusion despite adequate fluid loading and the use of vasopressor agents (weak recommendation, low quality of evidence).

Remarks: If initiated, vasopressor dosing should be titrated to an end point reflecting perfusion, and the agent reduced or discontinued in the face of worsening hypotension or arrhythmias.

After 2 h, her vital sign was improved to 112/60 mmHg–98 bpm–28 cpm–36.7 °C with CVP at 18 mmHg (Sat: 99%). O2 flow rate was decreased to 8 L/min, and norepinephrine infusion rate was decreased to 2 μg/min. O2 flow rate was further decreased to 4 L/min via nasal prong, and norepinephrine infusion was stopped. Her vital signs remained stable thereafter and her oxygen requirements gradually decreased. Dobutamine infusion was gradually tapered off. Later, her urine test for pneumococcus urine antigen was revealed to be positive. She was treated for 8 more hospital days with antibiotics. Her chest X-ray was improved during the hospital stay (Fig. 7.31).

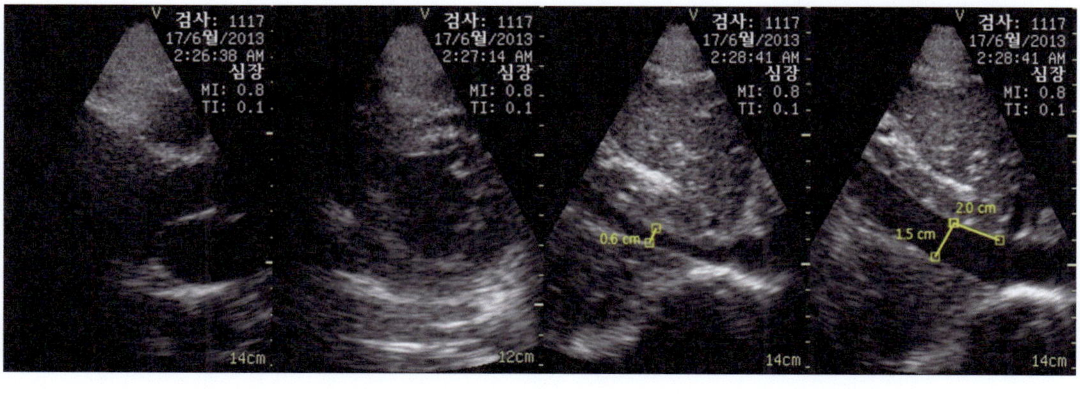

Fig. 7.31 Third bedside ultrasonography (HD 2) showing clear improvement in volume overload

7.7.1 Summary

This was a case of pneumococcal pneumonia septic shock. Since myocardial depression was combined, pulmonary edema and progression of hypoxemia were followed after initial fluid resuscitation. CVP was 24 mmHg and bedside echocardiography revealed dilated IVC diameter. Fluid was withheld and dobutamine was added to increase myocardial function. Her cardiac output was increased and norepinephrine was tapered. Pulmonary edema was improved with stabilization of vital sign. Bedside echocardiography and CVP provided important information to guide initial fluid administration and vasopressor and inotropic use in this patient.

7.8 A Septic Shock Case with Acute Cholangitis

A 79-year-old female came to the emergency department (ED) for abdominal pain. She was diagnosed with pancreatic head cancer with vascular invasion and peritoneal seeding diagnosed 6 months ago. She had biliary stent insertion procedure 5 months ago and was being treated with chemotherapy. Her initial vital signs were 77/59 mmHg–112 bpm–28 cpm–38.2 °C. The abdominal pain started with nausea and vomiting 2 days ago and, as time went by, the pain worsened. Physical examination revealed right upper quadrant tenderness.

Q. Please describe her current condition.

A. Infectious process should be considered because she is febrile. She can be in sepsis, because her initial qSOFA score was 2 (SBP 77 mmHg with increased respiratory rate at 28 cpm). Her blood pressure is very low at 77/59 mmHg. However, diagnosis of septic shock should be based on the response to adequate fluid resuscitation and serum lactate level.

Q. List your differential diagnoses and their rationales.

A. She has pancreatic cancer with prior history of biliary stent insertion for biliary obstruction. As she had right upper quadrant tenderness on physical examination without any other localizing sign, an infection involving hepatobiliary system should be at the first of the differential diagnosis list. Another possible explanation for her fever could be neutropenic fever because she was on chemotherapy until recently.

Q. Describe your initial management plan.

A. Clinically, she is suspected to be in sepsis and possibly in septic shock. SSC guideline recommends adequate fluid resuscitation, early administration of appropriate antibiotics, and source control in this condition. Fluid resuscitation should be guided by patients' volume status and empirical antibiotics should be administered within 1 h. Source control usually requires anatomic assessment of the patient which requires further evaluation (abdominal CT or sonography) in this patient (see page 68).

Because of initial RUQ pain and tenderness and underlying pancreatic head cancer with recent biliary stent procedure, the treating physician made initial presumptive diagnosis of acute cholangitis. After collection of culture specimens, the treating physician ordered piperacillin/tazobactam as initial empirical antibiotics to cover bacteria of biliary origin including pseudomonas.

Antibacterial Regimen for Acute Cholangitis

The most common bacteria isolated are as follows:

Gram negative

- *Escherichia coli* (most common, 25–50%) > Klebsiella (15–20%) > Enterobacter (5–10%).

Gram positive

- Enterococcus species (most common, 10–20%).

Anaerobes

- Bacteroides and Clostridia, usually present as a mixed infection.
- Rarely sole infecting organism, and not clear if they play a role in acute cholangitis (Nancy Misri Khardori, 2012).

Because of bacteriology as above, empiric antibiotic therapy for ascending cholangitis should include broad-spectrum parenteral antibiotics based upon the probable source of infection until culture results are available. The first-choice regimen of empiric therapy for gram negative and anaerobes was recommended to be monotherapy with a beta-lactam/beta-lactamase inhibitor such as piperacillin/tazobactam or combination third-generation cephalosporin such as ceftriaxone plus metronidazole.

Reference: Nancy Misri Khardori, Interventions in infectious disease emergencies, Medical clinics of north America, Medical Clinics of North America, Volume 96, Issue 6, Pages 1033–1272 (November 2012).

After fluid resuscitation as recommended by SSC guideline, her blood pressure increased, but was still low as 80/40 mmHg. Meanwhile, her initial laboratory results came out. The laboratory results can be summarized as leukocytosis, coagulopathy, metabolic acidosis (lactic acidosis), azotemia, and cholestasis. Her initial electrocardiogram showed no significant arrhythmia or ST-T change. Her chest X-ray showed no active lesion in both lung fields (Fig. 7.32).

Arterial blood gas analysis			CBC			Chemistry			Cardiac enzyme			Coagulation panel			Urinalysis		
pH	7.302		WBC	12,390	/μL	Na	142.9	mmol/L	CK	NA	ng/mL	PT	16	Seconds	WBC	5–9	/HPF
pCO2	22.9	mmHg	Hb	11.9	g/dL	K	3.5	mmol/L	CK-MB	NA	ng/mL	PT (INR)	1.42	INR	RBC	1–4	/HPF
pO2	70.6	mmHg	Hct	37.8	%	Cl	112.4	mmol/L	TnI	NA	pg/mL	aPTT	32.1	Seconds	Albumin	1+	
HCO3-	22.9	mmol/L	Platelet	55,000	/μL	TCO2	9.4	mmol/L				D-dimer	23.4	μg/mL	Nitrite	Negative	
Base excess	NA	mmol/L				BUN	25	mg/dL				Fibrinogen	NA	mg/dL	Bacteria	Many	
Lactate	10.53	mmol/L				Cr	1.76	mg/dL									
						AST	562	IU/L									
						ALT	316	IU/L									
						T.bil	3.5	mg/dL									
						ALP	127	IU/L									
						T.prot.	5.6	g/dL									
						Albumin	3.2	g/dL									

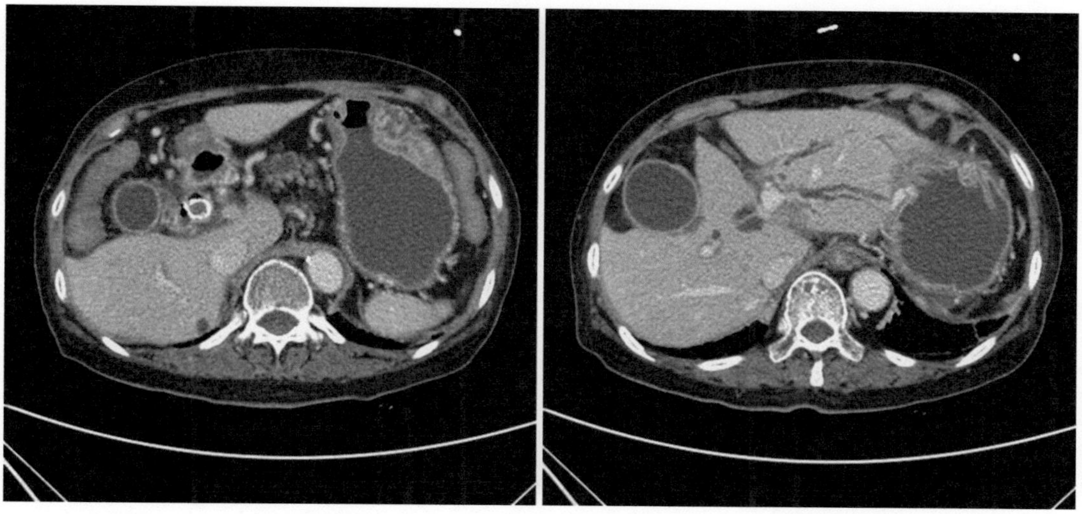

Fig. 7.32 Abdominal CT scan images of the patient. There were intrahepatic duct dilatation and GB distension with wall enhancement

Q. Her initial coagulation results were not normal. Do the findings indicate disseminated intravascular coagulation (DIC)?

A. Because DIC syndrome manifests in various forms by the etiology and disease process, there are no established diagnostic criteria and it should be diagnosed clinically. The International Society for Thrombosis and Hemostasis (ISTH) DIC scoring system provides objective measurement of DIC as follows:

Platelet count:
>100,000/μL = 0
50,000/μL–100,000/μL = 1
<50,000/μL = 2

Elevated fibrin-related markers such as soluble fibrin monomers and fibrin degradation products:
No increase = 0.
Moderate increase = 2.
Strong increase = 3.

Prolonged prothrombin time:
3 s or less = 0
>3 s but <6 s = 1
>6 s = 2

Fibrinogen level:
Greater than 100 mg/dL = 0.
<100 mg/dL = 1

Calculate score:
A total score ≥5 is compatible with overt DIC. It is recommended to repeat scoring daily.
Total score <5 suggests non-overt DIC, and the tests should be repeated in the next 1–2 days.

Reference: Levi M, Toh CH, Thachil J, Watson HG. Guidelines for the diagnosis and management of disseminated intravascular coagulation. Br J Haematol. 2009 Apr;145(1):24–33.

Q. Current SSC guideline recommends that a specific anatomic diagnosis of infection requiring emergent source control should be identified or excluded as rapidly as possible in patients with sepsis or septic shock. Please describe your initial plan for source control for this patient.

A. The patient is suspected of having acute cholangitis or other infections involving hepatobiliary system. The usual source control method for acute cholangitis is PTBD- or ERCP-guided biliary drainage. In case the patient has liver abscess, percutaneous drainage of the abscess should be arranged. In this case, abdominal enhanced CT was chosen over liver sonography for comprehensive assessment of whole abdominopelvic cavity.

During initial hemodynamic resuscitation, a total of 1.5 L of saline was administered intravenously. After the initial resuscitation, her blood pressure was 106/60 mmHg, and heart rate was 120. For further evaluation of her biliary system as well as to find other possible fever focus, the treating physician ordered an abdominal CT scan. The abdomen CT scan revealed intrahepatic duct dilatation and GB distension with wall enhancement which supports initial presumptive diagnosis of cholangitis (Fig. 7.33).

PTBD insertion was done after the resuscitation. However, her blood pressure gradually decreased. To maintain mean blood pressure over 65 mmHg, norepinephrine infusion was started and titrated up to 16 μg/min which increased her MBP to 80 mmHg (systolic/diastolic blood pressure was 114/62 mmHg). After 12 h of continuing treatment, the MBP remained stable at the rate of 12 μg/min of norepinephrine infusion which was gradually tapered thereafter.

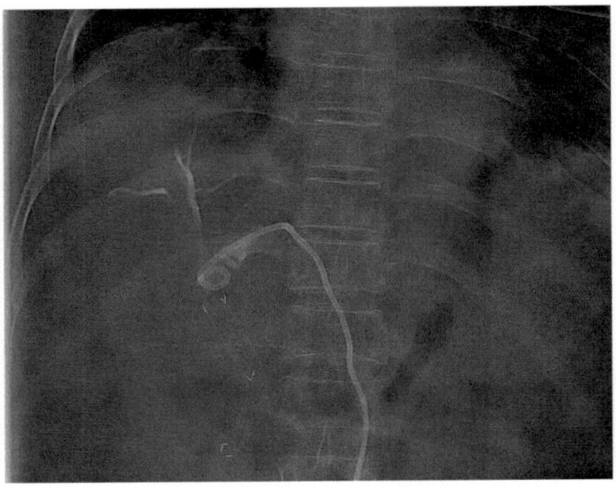

Fig. 7.33 PTBD insertion of the patient

Her blood and PTBD fluid cultures revealed ESBL-negative *K. pneumoniae* that was susceptible with cephalosporin, carbapenem, and aminoglycosides on fourth admission day. Therefore, antibiotic regimen was changed to ceftriaxone because current SCC guideline recommends that empiric antimicrobial therapy should be narrowed once pathogen identification and sensitivities are established and/or adequate clinical improvement is noted. Follow-up blood and PTBD fluid cultures were done after 1 week from the day of the first microbial cultures, and the result of blood and PTBD fluid cultures was negative. She was safely discharged to home with oral antibiotics at hospital day 10.

7.8.1 Summary

Cholangitis is one of the deadliest causes of sepsis. Prompt diagnosis, early antibiotics administration, and appropriate source control are critical as is true in other sepsis syndromes. Source control methods for biliary sepsis can be summarized as follows:

First of all, broad-spectrum antibiotics should be administered to the patient who is suspected of sepsis as soon as possible after microbial culture study. And it should be considered to take the imaging test first such as CT scan or ultrasound to make a decision whether or not to perform source control procedure. If there is an evidence of biliary tract obstruction such as biliary tract dilatation or tense gallbladder dilatation, it should be considered that the patients need urgent biliary decompression procedures. Especially, the patient who has persistent abdominal pain, hypotension despite adequate fluid resuscitation, fever greater than 39 °C, or mental confusion due to infection should be considered to receive urgent biliary decompression procedure such as ERCP, PTBD, or PTGBD appropriately.

7.9 A Septic Shock Case Due to *Klebsiella pneumoniae* Liver Abscess

A 72-year-old male patient came to the emergency department (ED) for visual loss on his left eye which began 1 day before the ED visit. His initial vital signs were 81/49 mmHg–79 bpm–18 cpm–38.7 °C.

Because the initial chief complaint of patient was visual loss, the physician focused on patient's eye problem and the initial decision was to arrange ophthalmologist examination. Patient was sent to the ophthalmology department at 1 h after ED arrival, and came back to the ED after staying for 3 h at the ophthalmology department for exam. Septic shock was recognized after the patient came back from the ophthalmology department; his blood pressure was 64/41 mmHg at that time.

Additional history finding revealed that the patient complained of myalgia for 5 days and watery diarrhea for 3 days. His physical examination revealed abdominal tenderness on right upper quadrant and pitting edema in both lower extremities.

Q. What has gone wrong with the initial management?

A. This patient should be suspected of having a sepsis because initial vital signs show low systolic blood pressure and increased body temperature. The treating physician did not notice the abnormalities and sent the patient to ophthalmological examination. The patient should be on monitor and getting appropriate management for suspected sepsis from the beginning. To avoid this mistake, routine implementation of a screening tool (e.g., qSOFA) to ED patients would be helpful.

After the recognition that patient is in septic shock state, which was 4 h past from ED arrival, the physician started to administer normal saline rapidly up to 2 L. His initial chest X-ray showed no active lung lesion and electrocardiogram showed no significant ST-T change nor arrhythmia. Routine laboratory tests were ordered including CRP and lactate to evaluate severity. After 2 h, his initial laboratory results came out as follows.

Arterial blood gas analysis			CBC			Chemistry			Cardiac enzyme			Coagulation panel			Urinalysis		
pH	7.34		WBC	8290	/μL	Na	132	mmol/L	CK	NA	ng/mL	PT (INR)	1.16	INR	WBC	NA	/HPF
pCO2	28	mmHg	Hb	12.9	g/dL	K	3.8	mmol/L	CK-MB	NA	ng/mL	aPTT	33.9	Seconds	RBC	NA	/HPF
pO2	86	mmHg	Hct	38.9	%	Cl	94	mmol/L	TnI	NA	pg/mL	D-dimer	NA	μg/mL	Albumin	NA	
HCO3-	NA	mmol/L	Platelet	49,000	/μL	TCO2	18	mmol/L							Nitrite	NA	
Base excess	−10.7	mmol/L				BUN	107	mg/dL							Bacteria	NA	
Lactate	NA	mmol/L				Cr	4.27	mg/dL									
						CRP	23	mg/L									
						AST	125	IU/L									
						ALT	99	IU/L									
						T.bil	1.5	mg/dL									
						ALP	73	IU/L									
						T.prot.	5.7	g/dL									
						Albumin	3.3	g/dL									

Bedside ultrasonography revealed hepatic mass in S6 area suspicious of liver abscess and collapsed inferior vena cava. Estimated ejection fraction of LV was above 60%.

Q. Does this patient have evidences of organ dysfunction?

A. The high creatinine level indicates azotemia and the high CRP level indicates underlying inflammatory processes in this patient. Organ dysfunction can be identified as an acute change in total SOFA score ≥2 points consequent to the infection. The baseline SOFA score can be assumed to be zero in patients not known to have preexisting organ dysfunction. We calculate SOFA score to evaluate the severity of organ dysfunction. The SOFA score was 7 (renal 3, cardiovascular 1, and hematologic 3). A SOFA score ≥2 reflects an overall mortality risk of approximately 10% in a general hospital population with suspected infection. The lactate level was 3.9, which is greater than the threshold for definition of shock (>2 mmol/L). However, we need to check the response to the fluid resuscitation to confirm septic shock (see page 60).

Until this time point, a total of 2300 mL of crystalloid was administered and central venous catheter was inserted. The Surviving Sepsis Campaign guideline recommends frequent reassessment of hemodynamic status to guide additional fluid administration. After initial fluid administration, his blood pressure increased, but was still low at 80/40 mmHg. To maintain mean blood pressure over 65 mmHg, norepinephrine was started and titrated up to 8 μg/min.

Q. Is this patient confirmed as septic shock?

A. According to the definition of the Sepsis-3, septic shock is a subset of sepsis in which underlying circulatory and cellular/metabolic abnormalities are profound enough to substantially increase mortality. This patient had persisting hypotension requiring vasopressors to maintain MAP ≥65 mmHg and having a serum lactate level >2 mmol/L despite adequate volume resuscitation. Therefore, this patient can be confirmed as septic shock. With these criteria, hospital mortality is reported to be in excess of 40%.

Because his initial physical examination showed right upper quadrant tenderness, and bedside ultrasound showed abscess like hepatic mass, an abdominal CT scan was taken to identify possible infection focus. Even though his creatinine level was 4.2 mg/dL, to evaluate abscess like lesion, physician at the site decided to order contrast abdomen CT (Fig. 7.34).

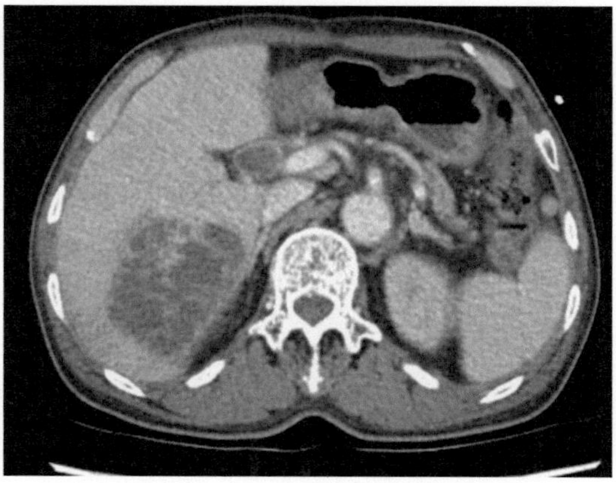

Fig. 7.34 A large abscess in the right posterior section of the liver

His abdomen CT revealed 8.5 cm pyogenic abscess in the right posterior section of the liver without a stone in his common bile duct (Fig. 7.34). He was assessed as septic shock due to pyogenic liver abscess with possible acute septic kidney injury.

The consulted ophthalmologist's diagnosis for the left eye visual loss was endogenous endophthalmitis due to metastatic infection. Considering that he had both liver abscess and endophthalmitis, *Klebsiella pneumoniae* liver abscess syndrome was highly suspicious. Biliary obstruction due to CBD stone may have played a significant role in this process.

Q. What is the *Klebsiella pneumoniae* liver abscess syndrome?

A. *Klebsiella pneumoniae* primary liver abscess (KLA) occurs in the absence of hepatobiliary disease and is almost always monomicrobial. Most cases have been reported from Asia or in patients of Asian origin. In addition to the manifestations typical of pyogenic liver abscess, such as fever, leukocytosis, right upper quadrant tenderness, and elevated liver enzymes, a minority of patients with primary KLA can develop metastatic infections at other sites. A high index of suspicion for metastatic spread to various other organs including the eye is necessary. Early detection of Klebsiella-associated endophthalmitis and prompt treatment with aggressive intravenous antibiotics may be the only method to salvage visual acuity and decrease the incidence of overall morbidity and mortality.

7.9.1 Progression

At 5 h after presentation, meropenem was started as initial empirical antibiotics after blood culture test. At the second hospital day, 1% vancomycin 1.0 mg/0.1 mL and 2.25% ceftazidime 2.25 mg/0.1 mL intraocular injections were done by the ophthalmology consultant. Despite the aggressive hemodynamic management, there was no urine output. So, continuous renal replacement therapy (CRRT) was started. Percutaneous catheter drainage (PCD) insertion in liver abscess was done. At hospital day 3, atrial fibrillation with rapid ventricular rate appeared and mental state of the patient was deteriorated to drowsy state. Intubation was done and mechanical ventilator support was started. At hospital day 4, his vital signs began to stabilize and norepinephrine was tapered off. At hospital day 5, culture reports came back. The *Klebsiella pneumoniae* (ESBL negative) was isolated in his blood and PCD fluid. Because current guidelines recommend empiric antimicrobial therapy be narrowed once pathogen is identified and sensitivities are established and/or adequate clinical improvement is noted; his antibiotics were stepped down to ceftriaxone 2 g bid (a dose for CNS infection) considering endophthalmitis. At hospital day 6, brain MRI imaging was done. There was no evidence of metastatic infection to CNS. The patient's overall conditions eventually got better and CRRT and mechanical ventilation were tapered off. The patient was transferred to general ward for further treatment.

7.9.2 Summary

This was a case of invasive syndrome of *Klebsiella pneumoniae* liver abscess. The patient came to the ED with visual loss and was found to have septic shock. Despite prompt assessment and aggressive treatment, he developed ARDS and acute kidney injury which made him to require CRRT and mechanical ventilation. *Klebsiella pneumoniae* is a well-known human pathogen, and recently a distinct invasive syndrome caused by *K. pneumoniae* serotypes K1 and K2 has been recognized in Southeast Asia. The syndrome is defined by the following criteria: (1) definite invasive syndrome: *Klebsiella pneumoniae* liver abscess with extrahepatic complications, especially CNS involvement, necrotizing fasciitis, or endophthalmitis and (2) probable invasive syndrome: *K. pneumoniae* liver abscess as the sole presenting clinical manifestation.

It is recommended that in patients with diabetes mellitus who present with *K. pneumoniae* bacteremia, endophthalmitis, meningitis, or other extrahepatic infections, especially those who are Asian or of Asian descent, a search for an occult liver abscess is indicated.

As current guidelines recommend, source control has utmost importance once initial hemodynamic stabilization and initiation of antibiotics are achieved. In cases where initial infection source is not clear, detailed history taking and physical examination as well as imaging workup such as CT can be revealing.

7.10 A Septic Shock Case Due to Acute Pyelonephritis

A 78-year-old woman being cared in a nursing hospital came to the emergency department (ED) for hypotension and altered mental status. She has been hemiplegic because of a stroke event 30 years ago. She was also treated for pulmonary tuberculosis 7 years ago. Her initial vital signs were 60/38 mmHg–106 bpm–18 cpm–39 °C. She developed fever and myalgia developed 2 days ago. Physical examination revealed left costovertebral angle tenderness (CVAT). There were no other historical clues to get because she was too drowsy for verbal communication. The Glasgow coma scale was E2M5V2. Bedside echocardiography examination was done and found collapsed IVC.

Q. Is she septic?

A. She had altered mental status and hypotension (SBP: 60 mmHg) which indicate possible sepsis according to qSOFA.

After fluid administration as recommended by the SCC guideline, her blood pressure increased, but was still low as 80/40 mmHg. Meanwhile, her initial laboratory test results came out.

Arterial blood gas analysis			CBC			Chemistry			Cardiac enzyme			Coagulation panel			Urinalysis		
pH	7.345		WBC	12,260	/μL	Na	136.4	mmol/L	CK	NA	ng/mL	PT (Sec)	12.9	Seconds	WBC	>100	/HPF
pCO2	32.7	mmHg	Hb	9.3	g/dL	K	4.4	mmol/L	CK-MB	4.7	ng/mL	PT (INR)	1.10	INR	RBC	5–9	/HPF
pO2	75.9	mmHg	Hct	27.2	%	Cl	102.8	mmol/L	TnI	0.066	pg/mL	aPTT	27.3	Seconds	Albumin	2+	
HCO3-	17.4	mmol/L	Platelet	135,000	/μL	TCO2	19.2	mmol/L	Pro-BNP	721.3	pg/dL	D-dimer	2.37	μg/mL	Nitrite	Positive	
Base excess	NA	mmol/L				BUN	38	mg/dL				Fibrinogen	467.5	mg/dL	Bacteria	Many	
Lactate	5.0	mmol/L				Cr	2.91	mg/dL									
						AST	28	IU/L									
						ALT	17	IU/L									
						T.bil	0.9	mg/dL									
						ALP	59	IU/L									
						T.prot.	6.2	g/dL									
						Albumin	3.6	g/dL									

Her initial laboratory findings indicated azotemia, lactic acidosis, and significant pyuria with bacteriuria. Her initial chest X-ray showed no active lesion in the lung compared with previous X-ray and electrocardiogram showed sinus tachycardia.

Q. What is your presumptive diagnosis of this patient and its rationale?

A. Considering CVAT, pyuria, and positive nitrite on her urinalysis, acute pyelonephritis should be considered as a primary diagnosis.

After obtaining specimens for blood and urinary cultures, meropenem was administered as the initial empirical antibiotics. The choice was based on the culture results of her previous admission when a drug-resistant bacterial strain (ESBL-positive *E. coli*) was cultured from her urine.

During the initial resuscitation, over 2 L of crystalloid fluid was administered. However, the patient remained hypotensive with BP of 92/30 mmHg. To maintain mean blood pressure over 65 mmHg, norepinephrine was started and titrated up to 8 μg/min. During initial resuscitation, the patient's oxygen saturation was decreased to 86%. Thus, follow-up chest X-ray was performed. Chest X-ray showed bilateral pleural effusion and pulmonary edema (Fig. 7.35).

Oxygen supply at the rate of 3 L/min was started using nasal prong. Although urine output had increased to 0.5 mg/kg/h, intravenous furosemide (20 mg) was administered to the patient because of her pulmonary edema.

To rule out other possible infection focuses as well as to find any evidence of complicated UTI, a non-contrast abdominal CT was taken. Contrast dye was not used because of the decreased renal function (Fig. 7.36).

Abdomen CT revealed left perirenal fat stranding with small amount of fluid collection which is

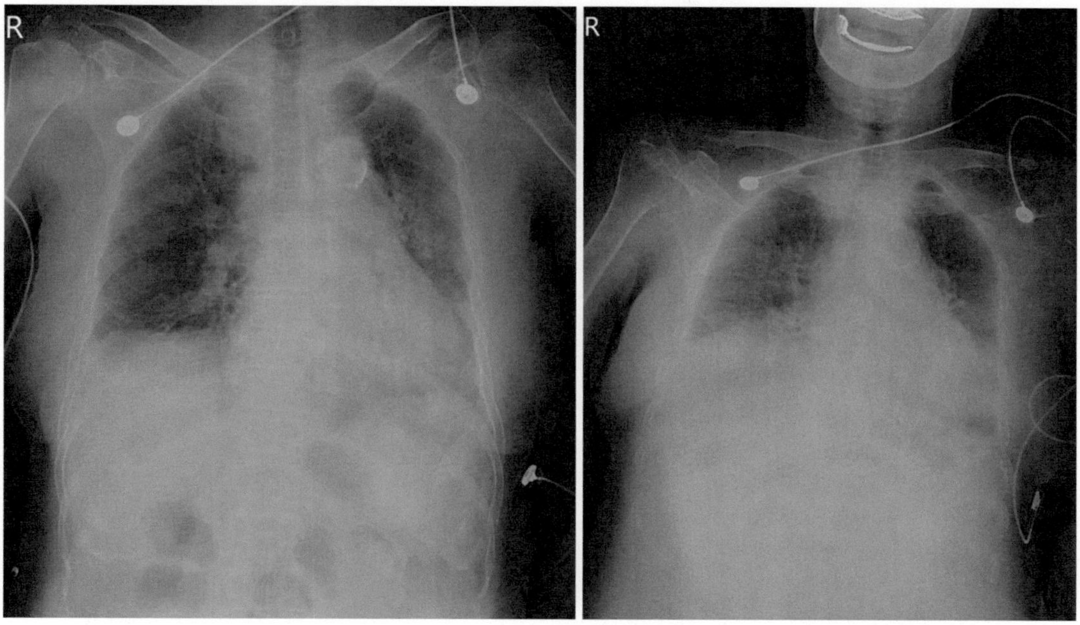

Fig. 7.35 Development of pleural effusion and pulmonary edema after fluid resuscitation

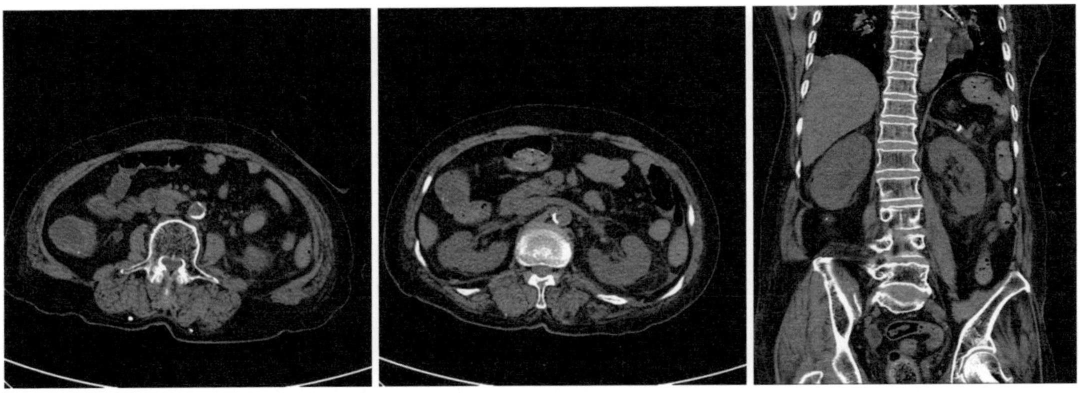

Fig. 7.36 Left: perirenal fat stranding with small amount of fluid collection suggesting acute pyelonephritis

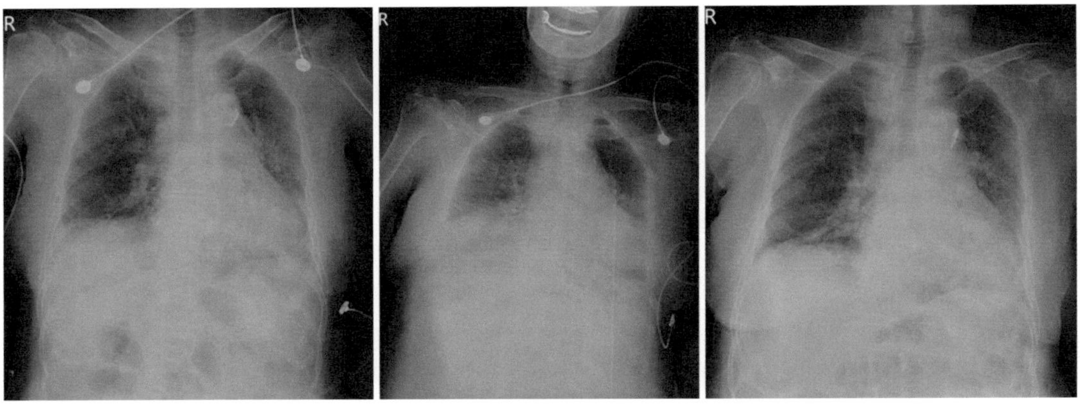

Fig. 7.37 Chest X-ray changes during fluid resuscitation. Left, 11 AM: no change; middle, 2 PM: increased pulmonary edema, bilateral atelectasis; right, next day 6 AM: decreased pulmonary edema, subsegmental atelectasis in the right lower lobe

> **Q. Would you recommend CT scan for this patient? What is your rationale if so?**
> A. Acute pyelonephritis is relatively a common infection. The grave presentation of the patient indicates that there could be complicated APN. Unenhanced abdominal CT can detect ureter stone and hydronephrosis both of which frequently warrant further evaluation and interventions for source control. Ultrasound can be an alternative choice.

suggestive of left pyelonephritis. Otherwise no other septic focus was found. Therefore, her ED diagnosis was made as septic shock caused by acute pyelonephritis.

After 24 h of treatment, mean blood pressure was maintained over 65 mmHg while maintaining norepinephrine infusion at 8 μg/min. Blood pressure was 128/50 mmHg, and heart rate was 120 bpm after 24 h from treatment start. Norepinephrine was tapered during the second hospital day. At the hospital day 2, the follow-up chest X-ray showed improvement of pulmonary edema and decreased extent of pleural effusion (Fig. 7.37).

Her blood and urine culture reports came out at hospital day 4. They were positive for ESBL(+) *E. coli* and the initial choice of antibiotics was maintained until her discharge. She was fully recovered and discharged at hospital day 11.

7.10.1 Summary

Acute pyelonephritis is a relatively common systemic infection. According to the report that Czaja CA wrote, overall annual rates are 15–17 cases per 10,000 females and 3–4 cases per 10,000 males Acute pyelonephritis develops in 20–30% of pregnant women (*Czaja CA, et al., Population-based epidemiologic analysis of acute pyelonephritis, Clin Infect Dis. 2007 Aug 1;45(3):273–80*). Delia Scholes also reported that sexual behaviors, patient and family history of UTI, and diabetes are associated with increased pyelonephritis risk (*Delia Scholes, et al., Risk factors associated with acute pyelonephritis in healthy women, Ann Intern Med. 2005 Jan 4;142(1):20–7*). In this patient, no significant risk factors for complicated pyelonephritis were found. However, although pyelonephritis responds well to antibiotics, it can turn into deadly infectious syndrome in some patients.

The antibiotics for complicated acute pyelonephritis include the following: cefepime, imipenem, meropenem, and piperacillin/tazobactam. This patient had previous history of ESBL(+) bacterial infection. The treating physician appropriately chose meropenem as the primary antibiotics. Because she was in shock and had been living in a nursing hospital and it means that she might have been exposed to drug-resistant bacterial strains. And that choice was right.

The initial fluid resuscitation had resulted in pulmonary edema which should have been avoided by multiple reassessment of volume status. Physicians treating shock should be vigilant on the patients' volume status to decide when to stop volume infusion and start to use vasopressors instead.

7.11 A Shock Case Due to Toxic Shock Syndrome

A 25-year-old male with tattoo on his back came to the emergency department (ED) with a 2-day history of myalgia, headache, chill, and cough. He was a nonsmoker and had no specific underlying disease before. His initial vital signs were 151/57 mmHg–140 bpm–23 cpm–38.7 °C. The tattooing had been done 3 days ago. On physical examination, there was diffuse erythroderma on his chest. At his back, where the tattoo was, redness, pustules, and tenderness were observed. One hour after the visit, he became drowsy with his vital signs of 73/36 mmHg–123 bpm–21 cpm–39.2 °C (Fig. 7.38).

After initial fluid resuscitation as recommended by SSC guideline, his blood pressure was increased, but still remained low as 80/40 mmHg. His initial chest X-ray showed no active lung lesion and electrocardiogram showed sinus tachycardia. Meanwhile, his initial laboratory test results came out.

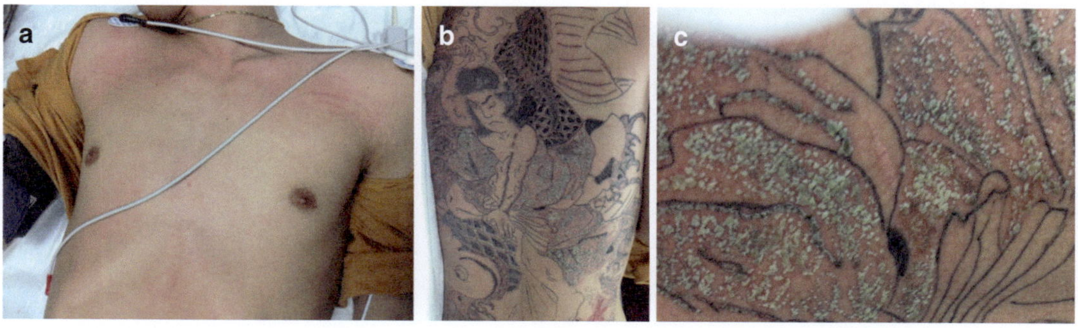

Fig. 7.38 The patient had diffuse erythroderma on his upper chest area (A). At his back, where the tattoo was, redness, pustules, and tenderness were observed

Arterial blood gas analysis			CBC			Chemistry			Cardiac enzyme			Coagulation panel			Urinalysis		
pH	7.45		WBC	25,940	/μL	Na	134	mmol/L	CK	NA	ng/mL	PT (%)	86	%	WBC	20–29	/HPF
pCO2	35	mmHg	Hb	13.8	g/dL	K	4.1	mmol/L	CK-MB	0.4	ng/mL	PT (INR)	1.12	INR	RBC	<1	/HPF
pO2	78	mmHg	Hct	38.7	%	Cl	94	mmol/L	TnI	0.001	pg/mL	aPTT	39.7	Seconds	Albumin	1+	
HCO3-	24.3	mmol/L	Platelet	154,000	/μL	TCO2	25	mmol/L				D-dimer	NA	μg/mL	Nitrite	Negative	
Base excess	NA	mmol/L				BUN	31	mg/dL				Fibrinogen	438	mg/dL	Bacteria	NA	
Lactate	2.2	mmol/L				Cr	1.77	mg/dL									
						AST	171	IU/L									
						ALT	170	IU/L									
						T.bil	1.3	mg/dL									
						ALP	74	IU/L									
						T.prot.	6.0	g/dL									
						Albumin	3.6	g/dL									

Q. What is your presumptive diagnosis and which evaluation steps are required to reach final diagnosis?

A. The patient is positive for two qSOFA criteria (SBP 73 mmHg, HR 123 cpm). Thus, he can be assumed to be in septic condition. Because he had high fever (≥38.9 °C), hypotension, elevated creatinine, skin rash (diffuse macular erythroderma on his chest and within tattoo), severe myalgia, drowsy mentality, and hepatic involvement (liver function test abnormality), azotemia, and coagulopathy, can also be assumed to be toxic shock syndrome. Blood, throat, or cerebrospinal fluid cultures are needed for final diagnosis and close observation for desquamation on his skin.

After 45 min of visiting the ED, antibiotics (vancomycin 1 g bid + clindamycin 4 mL tid + ceftriaxone 2 g qd) were started. Then immunoglobulin (monomeric purified polyspecific immunoglobulin G) was injected by intravenous route. During initial hemodynamic stabilization process, over 2 L of crystalloid was administered and central venous catheter was inserted. Follow-up vital signs were 98/57 mmHg–116 bpm–19 cpm–39.1 °C. To maintain mean blood pressure over 65 mmHg, norepinephrine infusion was started and titrated up to 12 μg/min.

Q. Why these antibiotics were chosen?

A. Broad-spectrum antibiotics should be administered as soon as possible in all suspected cases of TSS, preferably following collection of blood and other samples for culture. Current recommendations for empiric antibiotic treatment of suspected sepsis advocate the use of flucloxacillin and a third-generation cephalosporin. In settings where the rate of methicillin-resistant *S. aureus* (MRSA) is high, initial cover should include vancomycin. In our case, we decided to use antibiotics (ceftriaxone 2 g once daily + vancomycin 1 g twice a day + clindamycin 4 mL three times a day) to cover both *S. aureus* (including MRSA) and *S. pyogenes*.

Clindamycin has multiple activities that make it potentially useful as an adjunctive treatment in TSS. Clindamycin is a bacteriostatic lincosamide with efficacy unaffected by bacterial growth phase or inoculum size. Clindamycin has been shown to inhibit toxin production by both *S. aureus* and *S. pyogenes*. These include the ability to overcome the "Eagle effect," inhibition of superantigen toxin production, better tissue penetration and longer post-antibiotic effect than penicillin, and potentiation of phagocytosis. Clindamycin can also reduce bacterial superantigen toxin production through the inhibition of transcription of exoprotein genes, thereby potentially interrupting any ongoing stimulation of the inflammatory cascade. Clindamycin should not be used alone because it is only bacteriostatic rather than bactericidal and because of reports of rising resistance and improved outcomes have been reported with the combined use of a beta-lactam antibiotic and clindamycin.

Q. What is the role of immunoglobulin in TSS?

A. In TSS, the adjunctive use of intravenous immunoglobulin (IVIg) is supported on a theoretical basis by its anti-inflammatory and immunomodulatory properties, and on the evidence from many studies. IVIg contains mainly monomeric purified polyspecific immunoglobulin G (IgG) and a smaller fraction comprising other immunoglobulin isotypes and additional immunological components. The beneficial anti-inflammatory and immunomodulatory activities of IVIg when used in TSS are thought to include the facilitation of antigen recognition, activation of the innate immune system, and counteraction of superantigen toxin activity by neutralizing antibody and blockade T-cell activation by staphylococcal and streptococcal superantigens.

Diagnosis of Staphylococcal Toxic Shock Syndrome Clinical Case Definition

1. Fever ≥38.9 °C.
2. Hypotension—systolic blood pressure ≤90 mm Hg for adults.
3. Rash—diffuse macular erythroderma.
4. Desquamation—1–2 weeks after onset of illness, especially of palms and soles.
5. Multisystem involvement—three or more of the following:
   (a) Gastrointestinal—vomiting or diarrhea at the onset of illness.
   (b) Muscular—severe myalgia or elevated creatine phosphokinase.
   (c) Mucous membranes—vaginal, oropharyngeal, conjunctival hyperemia.
   (d) Renal—blood urea nitrogen or creatinine twice upper limit of normal.
   (e) Hepatic—total bilirubin twice upper limit of normal.
   (f) Hematological—platelets ≤100/μL.
   (g) CNS—disorientation or alterations in consciousness without focal neurological signs.
6. Negative results on the following tests:
   (a) Blood, throat, or cerebrospinal fluid culture (blood culture may be positive for *S. aureus*).
   (b) Rise in titer to Rocky Mountain spotted fever, leptospirosis, or measles.

   Case classification.

   *Probable: case with five of the six clinical findings described

   *Confirmed: case with all six of the clinical findings described.

Treatment of Staphylococcal Toxic Shock Syndrome

1. Aggressive fluid replacement with normal saline to treat hypotension.
2. The prompt administration of appropriate antibiotics: In cases in which the causative organism is unknown, the antibiotic regimen should cover both *S. aureus* (including MRSA if indicated) and *S. pyogenes*.
   - Broad-spectrum antibiotics (flucloxacillin + third-generation cephalosporin) + clindamycin
     ~Then changes ~.
   - Cloxacillin or nafcillin or cefazolin + clindamycin (MSSA if indicated).
   - Vancomycin or teicoplanin (MRSA if indicated) + clindamycin.
3. Consider use of intravenous immunoglobulin (IVIg) in patients whom no clinical response within the first 6 h of aggressive supportive therapy:
   IV Ig G [high dose (1–2 g/kg) on day 1 followed by subsequent doses of 0.5 g/kg on days 2 and 3].
4. Source control (for staphylococcal TSS, source control may include removal of the tampon or drainage of a surgical site infection).
5. Extracorporeal membrane oxygenation (ECMO) and supportive management.

7.11.1 Progression

After 1 day, methicillin-sensitive *Staphylococcus aureus* was isolated from the skin wound culture. No organism was isolated from blood culture. Antibiotics were changed to cefazolin + clindamycin. Norepinephrine was tapered to 4 μg/min. After 2 days, norepinephrine was tapered off. He was transferred to general ward and antibiotic therapy was maintained until discharge. After 5 days, characteristic skin desquamation began at back, finger, and toe area which supports the initial diagnosis of TSS. After 14 days, he was discharged home (Fig. 7.39).

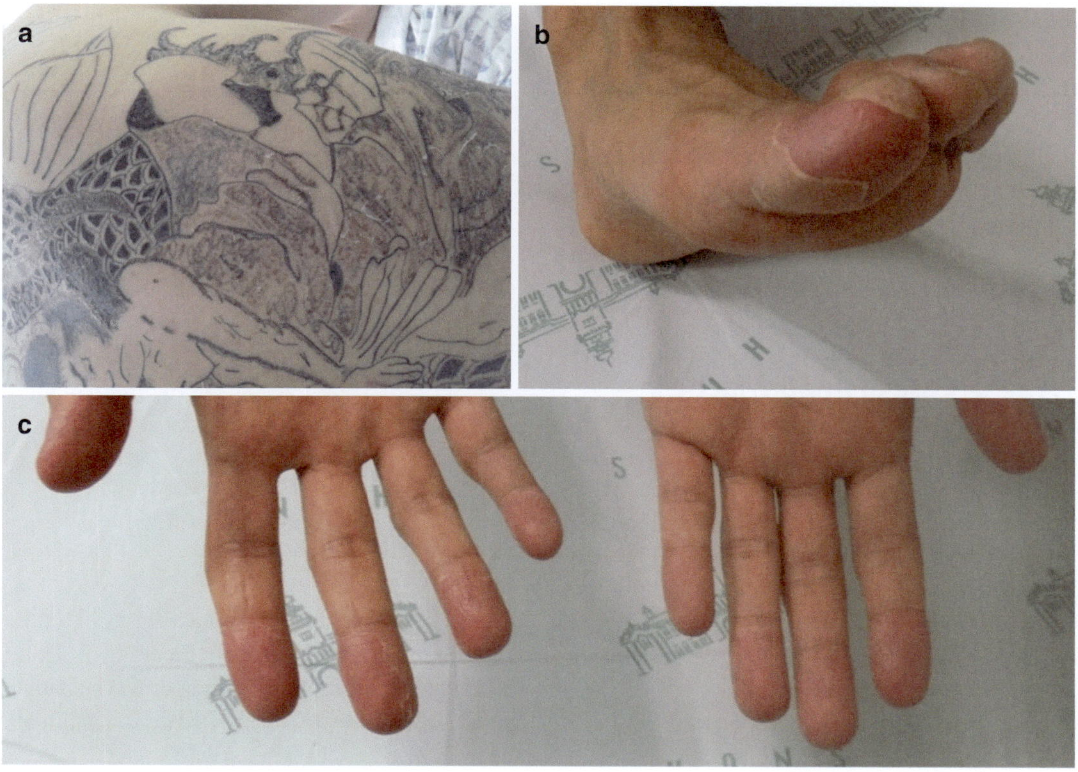

Fig. 7.39 Desquamation of skin occurred within tattoo on back (**a**), left toe (**b**), and both fingers (**c**) observed at outpatient department visit

7.11.2 Summary

This was a classic case of a toxic shock syndrome due to methicillin-sensitive *Staphylococcus aureus*. Patient came to the ED with fever, myalgia, and skin rash after tattooing. Toxic shock syndrome (TSS) is an acute, multisystem, toxin-mediated illness, often resulting in multi-organ failure. It is caused by toxin-producing strains of *Staphylococcus aureus* and *Streptococcus pyogenes* (group A streptococcus). In this case, the treating physician promptly identified possible TSS case and administered appropriate antibiotic regimen early, while initial hemodynamic resuscitation process was still ongoing. The readers should remember that this prompt assessment of patient and early administration of antibiotics are critical in the management of septic shock.

7.12 A Case of Anaphylactic Shock

A 74-year-old man (75 Kg) with underlying hypertension came to the emergency department (ED) for persistent vomiting. His blood pressure and pulse rate were 110/60 mmHg and 66 bpm. He had skin rash in face and extremity. He had swollen face and lip. But his respiration was 18 cpm and he had no dyspnea.

About 20 min before the symptom onset, patient took his wife's painkiller (Aceclofenac 100 g) for headache. He had no known allergies. On the physical examination, his lung sound was normal without wheezing or stridor.

Q. What is your presumptive diagnosis and its rationales?

A. He had persistent vomiting and skin rash after taking the nonsteroidal anti-inflammatory drug (NSAID). They involve both cutaneous and gastrointestinal system after exposure to likely allergen. Although he had no previous history of allergic reaction, anaphylaxis should be included in the differential diagnoses because of the definition of anaphylaxis criteria 1 or 2. Blood tests are not necessary for the diagnosis of anaphylaxis. However, measuring serum tryptase and histamine may help to distinguish anaphylaxis from other diseases with similar symptoms. Similarly, chest X-ray and electrocardiogram can also be helpful.

His chest X-ray showed no active lesion in the lung or significant cardiomegaly. Electrocardiogram showed no significant arrhythmia or ST-T change. Initial laboratory tests showed no significant abnormalities.

Arterial blood gas analysis			CBC			Chemistry			Cardiac enzyme			Coagulation panel			Urinalysis		
pH	7.313		WBC	7450	/μL	Na	139	mmol/L	CK	68	ng/mL	PT (INR)	1.01	INR	WBC	1–4	/HPF
pCO2	43.6	mmHg	Hb	13.4	g/dL	K	3.5	mmol/L	CK-MB	1.5	ng/mL	aPTT	23.6	Seconds	RBC	1–4	/HPF
pO2	63.4	mmHg	Hct	39.6	%	Cl	102.8	mmol/L	TnI	<0.01	pg/mL	D-dimer	1.13	μg/mL	Albumin	1+	
HCO3-	21.6	mmol/L	Platelet	170,000	/μL	TCO2	20.2	mmol/L							Nitrite	Negative	
Base excess	−4.6	mmol/L				BUN	17	mg/dL							Bacteria	NA	
Lactate	5.31	mmol/L				Cr	1.45	mg/dL									
						AST	31	IU/L									
						ALT	28	IU/L									
						T.bil	0.7	mg/dL									
						ALP	45	IU/L									
						T.prot.	6.0	g/dL									
						Albumin	3.8	g/dL									

Q. What is your initial management plan?

A. 1:1000 (1 mg/mL) epinephrine 0.01 mg/kg should be injected by the intramuscular route in the mid-anterolateral thigh as soon as possible. In this case, 0.5 mg IM injection would be appropriate because the maximum dose of epinephrine IM injection for anaphylaxis is 0.5 mg in adults.

Although H1-antihistamines cannot inhibit the release of mediators from mast cells and basophils, it can relieve itching, flushing, urticaria, angioedema, and nasal and eye symptoms. Thus chlorpheniramine 10 mg or diphenhydramine 25–50 mg can be administered intravenously.

Glucocorticoids can switch off transcription of a multitude of activated genes that encode pro-inflammatory proteins. They can potentially relieve protracted anaphylaxis symptoms and prevent biphasic anaphylaxis, even though these effects have never been proven. Therefore, glucocorticoids are not lifesaving in initial hours of an anaphylactic episode, but they can be considered as second-line medications. Hydrocortisone 200 mg or methylprednisolone 1 mg/kg can be administered intravenously.

His symptoms were completely resolved after 0.5 mg IM injection of epinephrine. The patient wanted to be discharged home.

Q. Will you discharge the patient?

A. Biphasic anaphylaxis can occur in about 5–10% of anaphylaxis patients. Patients should be monitored for at least 4 h and, if necessary, up to 24 h.

Two hours later, tachycardia (112 bpm) with desaturation (SpO2 at 90%) developed. Patient had dyspnea and his blood pressure was 78/40 mmHg. EKG monitoring showed sinus tachycardia with no ST-segment abnormality. There was no evidence of urticaria, flush, or facial edema.

Q. What happened and what is the appropriate treatment?

A. The patient had respiratory (dyspnea, hypoxemia) and cardiovascular system (hypotension) involvement after complete resolution of initial anaphylactic reaction without re-exposure to the trigger. Therefore, the presumptive diagnosis is biphasic anaphylaxis.

- The treatment of biphasic anaphylaxis is the same as the anaphylaxis.
- A 1:1000 (1 mg/mL) epinephrine 0.01 mg/kg should be injected by the intramuscular route in the mid-anterolateral thigh as soon as possible.
- Give high-flow supplemental oxygen (6–8 L/min) by face mask. Place patient on the back, or in a position of comfort if there is respiratory distress.
- Give 1–2 L of 0.9% (isotonic) saline rapidly.

Ten minutes later, dyspnea and hypoxemia improved but the patient was still hypotensive (80/42 mmHg).

Q. What should be the next step?

A. A repeat dose of 1:1000 (1 mg/mL) epinephrine 0.01 mg/kg should be the choice. One can also consider vasopressors such as dopamine, norepinephrine, phenylephrine, or vasopressin. Administration of glucagon should also be considered when the patient is taking beta-adrenergic blocker or other medications that interfere with epinephrine effect. In case of cardiac arrest, the ECMO should be considered early in patients unresponsive to traditional resuscitative measures, before irreversible ischemic acidosis develops.

Patient's blood pressure gradually increased to 108/57 mmHg after another epinephrine injection. He was admitted to the short-stay unit for 24-h observation. Until the next day, there was no recurrent anaphylaxis. He was discharged with an Epi-pen prescription.

7.12.1 Summary

In this case, the patient with anaphylaxis involving cutaneous and gastrointestinal system was safely managed with early recognition of anaphylaxis. The most important component in the initial management of anaphylactic shock is giving epinephrine. Physicians should also recognize that anaphylaxis may not appear life threatening initially without respiratory or cardiovascular symptoms. During the observation period, he had lethal biphasic anaphylaxis and was appropriately managed with oxygen supply, epinephrine injection, and fluid resuscitation. The flowchart below points out a prompt diagnostic approach and management of anaphylaxis.

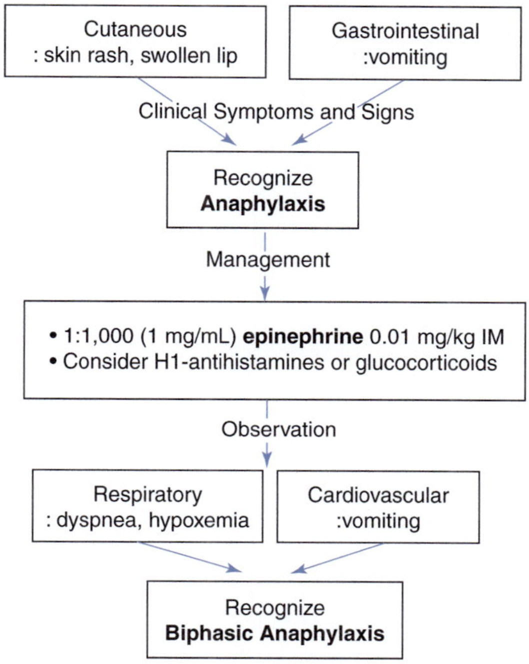

MIX
Papier aus verantwortungsvollen Quellen
Paper from responsible sources
FSC® C105338

If you have any concerns about our products,
you can contact us on
ProductSafety@springernature.com

In case Publisher is established outside the EU,
the EU authorized representative is:
Springer Nature Customer Service Center GmbH
Europaplatz 3, 69115 Heidelberg, Germany

Printed by Libri Plureos GmbH
in Hamburg, Germany